GW01191183

Also by Angelia Hulsey Carpenter

First Step in Missions, Volume 15
published by Woman's Missionary Union,
Birmingham, AL

From One Survivor ...
to Another ...
to Another ...
to Another

A Breast Cancer Survivor's Handbook

Jean Hulsey and Angelia Hulsey Carpenter

CROSSBOOKS
PUBLISHING

CrossBooks™
A Division of LifeWay
1663 Liberty Drive
Bloomington, IN 47403
www.crossbooks.com
Phone: 1-866-879-0502

First published by CrossBooks 6/06/2013

ISBN: 978-1-4627-2803-9 (sc)
ISBN: 978-1-4627-2804-6 (e)

Printed in the United States of America.

Jean

I dedicate my contribution to this book to my children: Angelia, Janice, Cindy, and Kent. Their encouragement and presence kept me going.

Angelia

I dedicate my contribution to my husband, Tom. There is no one else I wanted to take on this journey with me! And to Mom.......you showed me faith and true dependence on God for all your needs and how to take this journey called cancer.

CONTENTS

Foreword ix

Preface. xiii

Acknowledgement xvii

Introduction xxi

Chapter 1   I Have What?!. 1

Chapter 2   Educating Yourself 13

Chapter 3   The Big C—Chemotherapy 27

Chapter 4   Where Did I Put My Wig? 51

Chapter 5   Radiation and the Tattoos. 61

Chapter 6   Back for more Chemo 81

Chapter 7   Hallelujah Day!. 111

Chapter 8   Because of the Journey 121

Chapter 9   The Co-Survivor/Caretaker's
                    Perspective. 131

Scriptures that Encouraged Us. 147

Epilogue. 149

FOREWORD

Angelia and I first met in 1989 when we were both working for the Tennessee Baptist Convention. I met her mother during the early 90's as well. What I remember about them both is their sense of humor and solid faith in God. Angelia and I became fast friends and shared many wonderful years together before her life's journey took her away from middle Tennessee.

Who would've ever known that many years later we'd share another common path…cancer? When Jean (Angelia's mother) was diagnosed with breast cancer, soon after her husband was killed in a car accident, I remember grieving and praying for her. I stood from a distance and watched as her children rallied to her support, and am personally encouraged today by her strength and health. If she can conquer her cancer, perhaps I can conquer mine.

Then when Angelia was diagnosed my heart was broken. We were far too young to have to deal with serious life-threatening diseases like cancer. As I prayed, I watched and again stood amazed as Angelia's solid faith demonstrated itself in her email updates. I am so grateful that she took the time to journal her way through her battle. We were able to visit with one another briefly at the airport in Alexandria, Louisiana during the "no hair" stage of her treatment and I was impressed with the joy that radiated from her; joy that was real—not like the wig she "put on" to go out.

Little did I know then that I would be taking a similar journey in the near future. While I haven't fought breast cancer, I am fighting colon cancer. My journey is somewhat different, but as I read this book I could identify with so much of what Angelia and Jean experienced. I love their candor and their details. Cancer can be a scary thing, and not knowing (or not understanding) the medical procedures just makes it that much more frightening. Angelia and Jean do a great job of telling you in layman's terms what to expect from scans, surgery, chemotherapy and all the other things that we experience in the good fight.

But even more than the comfort they bring to their readers through their explanations of medical terms and procedures, I appreciate their honesty in describing how the cancer affected them emotionally and spiritually. Sometimes we feel like we have to be superhuman and somehow use this terrible time to be a model Christian. I cannot tell you how much comfort I found in reading that Jean (this great woman of incredible faith) cried at night. I cried at night, almost every night, during the weeks of my own chemo treatments and wondered if my tears somehow diluted my faith. But when I read her confession about her own tears I realized that I was okay, that God was still God and that He makes allowances for salty tears during chemo treatment.

The other part of this book that I really appreciate is the invitation to write in it. This book is more than a retelling of Jean and Angelia's story, it's your story too. As you read their stories, be encouraged to write your own for the day will come when God will use your story to encourage someone else.

I've not been brave (or clear minded) enough to write my own reflections of my cancer journey yet. But the year I was diagnosed, I wrote *Spiritual Warfare for Women* (Bethany House Publishers), and in that book I wrote this statement that I've found to be absolutely true:

Every attack of the Enemy brings with it a divine invitation from the hand (and heart) of God to know (by experience) what love does.

As you read *From One Survivor to Another...to Another...to Another...* you will find that statement to be true in your life too. I would imagine that you are reading these words because you, or someone you love, has heard the words, "It's cancer." If that's the case, read on and smile—for you're not the first one to take this trip and I promise God has riches He is eager to reveal to you along the way.

Leighann McCoy
Pray All the Way Ministries
Prayer & Women's Minister at Thompson Station Church, Thompson Station, TN

PREFACE

My mother, Jean Hulsey, was diagnosed with breast cancer in March 2005, nine short months after my father was killed in a car accident. My siblings (two sisters and a brother) and I met in Missouri for the day of the lumpectomy. We handle these situations with humor to cover our fear and anxiety. The morning of surgery we rose early to go with mom to the hospital wearing bandages on the right side of our chest. Even my brother and brother-in-law! We drew many stares and smiles.

We walked on this journey with mom. Probably more so because daddy wasn't by her side physically. He was always very protective and shielded us from bad news. Once we didn't even know she was having a partial hysterectomy until the surgery was over!

My far away sister, Cindy, and I went to mom's as often as our work schedules allowed, to take her to the doctor, to chemo, and later radiation. My sister, Janice, who lived nearby, usually took her to all of these appointments. Kent, who lives in Springfield, often met Mom and Janice at the cancer center for her treatments. I was always amazed by Mom's spirit, her outlook, and her faith that guided her on this journey. During her treatments she took a trip to South Carolina (the first grandchild's high school graduation), to England (for an already scheduled conference and tour), to Iowa (for a historical convention meeting), and repainted her family room as well as teaching Sunday School every week she was in town.

Mom often said there were things she couldn't remember or wish she had written down. I served as the family communications coordinator during this time and relayed information and news to friends and family through notes and e-mail. People often responded by e-mail and I forwarded that encouragement to her. When her treatments were finished I gave her a scrapbook with all the e-mails sent and received, mementoes (including the bandages we wore)! Having the scrapbook helped her remember the little things and reminded her of all the support and prayers during her cancer journey.

When asked before going into surgery, by one of the nurses, if she was nervous, Mom's reply was, "No, I figure this is a win, win situation. If I make it through the surgery and everything is fine I get to be with my children. If I don't, I get to be home with the Lord." Her strength has been an inspiration to us all. She truly understands the Scripture, "Do not be anxious about anything, but in every situation, by prayer and petition, with thanksgiving, present your requests to God. And the peace of God, which transcends all understanding, will guard your hearts and your minds in Christ Jesus (Philippians 4:6-7, NIV)" through experience not just head knowledge.

When I (Angelia) was diagnosed with breast cancer in October 2009 the first thing I did was go and buy a journal. I told Tom, my husband, "I want to write my feelings—grief, anger, praises—down. On the really bad days I can look back and see how God worked in my life on this journey." Tom and I prayed that God would use this pause in our lives as a ministry opportunity.

ACKNOWLEDGEMENT

Words are not adequate to begin to express our appreciation for each and every person who walked on this journey with us. Cancer doesn't affect one person. It affects and involves a multitude of people. We would like to thank the following for being a part of our journey in a variety of ways.

Jean Hulsey

The medical staff of St. John's Medical Center in Lebanon, MO—Dr. Ron Glass, Dr. Frank Roam, Dr. Karen Tabb and nurses

The medical staff of Whiteside (Chub O'Reilly) Cancer Center in Springfield, MO—Dr. Patrick Gomez, Dr. Anderson, Dr. Lavanya Tiriveedhi, Dr. Helen Kim, Barbara, Phyllis, Debbie, Jennifer and nurses

Ozark Cancer Research—Marsha

First Baptist Church, Lebanon, MO family who took me to treatments and provided meals

My children—Angelia & Tom Carpenter, Janice & Floyd Barnes, Cindy & Danny Smith, and Kent & Carrie Hulsey

My extended family—grandchildren, sisters, nieces, nephews

Peggy McVay—Linda's Hair Design, Lebanon, MO

First Baptist Church, Simpsonville, SC

Youth and leaders of Community Baptist Church, Waterloo, IA

The Woman's Missionary Union, SBC family

Friends from various stages of my life who sent notes, called, and e-mailed

Angelia Hulsey Carpenter

The staff of Christus St. Francis Cabrini Breast Center, Surgery Center, and Cancer Center in Alexandria, LA— Chris, Dr. David McCoy, Dr. Lawrence Menache, Angie Roberts, Dr. Ulla Ule, Kasey Gill, Janet Bonnette, Janet, Carolyn, Linda, Nicole, Lora, Jacey, Christy, Tina, Suzanne, Rebecca, Cindy, Chris, Ann

Kingsville Baptist Church, Ball, LA family for rides to treatment and meals

My family—Tom (my husband), Jean Hulsey (mom), Janice & Floyd Barnes, Cindy & Danny Smith, Kent & Carrie Hulsey

My extended family—cousins, in-laws, nieces, nephews

Melissa—JC Penney's Hair Salon, Alexandria, LA

Peggy McVay—Linda's Hair Design, Lebanon, MO

First Baptist Church, Simpsonville, SC

The Woman's Missionary Union, SBC family

Friends from various stages of my life who sent notes, flowers, gifts, called, and e-mailed
Shaun Martin, graphic designer
Janice Barnes, photographer

INTRODUCTION

Breast cancer is not exactly the kind of thing you want to have or share with anyone. Yet Mom and I did and do share this unique bond. We were diagnosed four years apart. There were many parallels in our treatments. For me (Angelia) it was good to have someone who had 'been there, done that, have the scars' to call and ask questions of.

As you read the story of our breast cancer journeys we pray they will be an encouragement to you, a source of knowing you aren't in the fight alone. At the end of each chapter will be three things: *Survivor tips*—what are some things we did to make this journey a little easier; *Co-survivor in action*—a list of things a co-survivor can do for the patient AND the family to minister to them; and *My thoughts and feelings*—an opportunity for you to begin recording your own feelings and thoughts. These lists are not at all exhaustive. Each cancer patient's needs and situation are different. We pray this will be a resource that you can pass on *from one survivor to another...to another....to another.*

Chapter 1

I HAVE WHAT?!

Jean

The year 2005 became a journey I never expected. In February, my daughter Janice and I traveled from Missouri to Iowa for a wedding. After the rehearsal Janice and I returned to the motel and began preparing for bed. All week I had had a pain. While brushing my teeth I leaned over the sink and pushed on the spot to relieve the pain. I felt the lump. From that point on I was almost sure it was cancer. I had the worst pain—unusual and persistent. It felt like someone was consistently stabbing me. I had always heard there wasn't pain when it was cancer. But even with the uncertainty and pain there was such peace.

Returning home on Monday I made a visit to the medical doctor. The whirlwind began—mammogram, ultrasound, visit to the surgeon for a biopsy. Within four days the results of the biopsy came back—it was an aggressive stage 2 breast cancer. My tumor was 2 cm. My Sunday School class knew I was waiting for the biopsy results. Two of the class members, Faye Dean and Hazel, came by the house shortly after I got the results. They sat at the kitchen table with me and had a cup of tea. I don't remember the conversation but I remember their presence and being there supporting me. I was stunned by the diagnosis, even though I think I knew it was cancer all along.

There was an experience during this time that helped me have the strength for the journey. Having lost my husband in an auto accident, just nine months before the diagnosis, I felt the loss deeply because of the lack of Lonney's presence. We were always there for each other but this time when I came from having my mammogram done, he was not there to greet me. Praying one night I asked God, "WHY, why did I have to go through this without Lonney?" The answer came clearly as if God was standing in front of me speaking out loud, "If Lonney was here you wouldn't depend on Me." From that point on there was peace and strength. God is sufficient!

The surgeon said that all options were mine— lumpectomy (removing the lump) or mastectomy (removing the breast). I chose lumpectomy. An appointment was made with the oncologist, Dr. Gomez. The lumpectomy was scheduled for March 24, 2005. My children—three daughters, one son, and one son-in-law came to the hospital wearing bandages on their right breasts in my honor. When asked, before going into surgery, by one of the nurses if I was nervous, I replied, "No, I figure this is a win, win situation. If I make it through the surgery and everything is fine I get to be with my children. If I don't, I get to go home to be with the Lord."

The lump was removed and I was sent directly home. I am very susceptible to medication and anesthesia so it takes quite awhile to become lucid. For two or three days grogginess was my companion. Two of my daughters, Cindy and Angelia, became nurses. They documented inputs, outputs, medication, sleeping habits. Because I was sent home with minimal instruction they wrote down everything they did.

I had a follow-up visit with Dr. Gomez. There was not enough tissue, around the lump, removed to give an accurate picture of the extent of the cancer. Another surgery was scheduled to remove additional tissue. After the healing it was time to schedule chemo and radiation.

Angelia

The morning of September 18, 2009, I went to Christus St. Frances Cabrini Hospital for a 6-month follow-up mammogram in my left breast because of suspicions the doctor had over a year ago. (I'd been doing mammograms every 6 months.) The nurse, Chris, told me it was about time for my yearly mammogram so she was going to call the doctor to get orders to do both breasts.

They took pictures several times of my right breast and then two ultrasounds—one with the mammographer and one with a doctor. The nurse showed me the film and I saw the white spot. As I lay on the table looking at the ceiling I thought, *"They need pictures on the ceiling so one's imagination doesn't go wild."* Then I began to think of all the things I would have to reschedule if I had cancer. I knew there was a strong possibility given our family history—mom, her sister, daddy's sister. Dr. Raj felt it was benign, told me to continue self-exams and come back in three months. If it was still there in three months they would do a biopsy. I had to ask him where to check specifically. I saw the film and you could definitely see what they were looking at. They found NOTHING in the left breast!!

During the afternoon the radiologist called back to tell me my family doctor was going to call. Immediately my heart jumped into my throat and my stomach started turning. Dr. Piland called and said the consensus was to go ahead and schedule a biopsy. Things weren't as clear on the sonogram as the mammogram so they felt it best to do the biopsy now instead of waiting three months. He then asked me who my surgeon was. I don't know about you but I usually look for a church home, dentist, hairdresser, grocery store, etc when I move to a new town. Up to this point I had no need for a surgeon. Dr. Piland suggested Dr. McCoy. He was going to make the appointment for me and call me back.

Tom, my husband, and I went to see Dr. McCoy on Tuesday, September 29th. He explained how the biopsy would be performed and both sides of the diagnosis—benign or malignant. Biopsies were done on Tuesdays and Fridays. Even though we had plans to go to Houston that coming weekend I was ready to schedule the biopsy for that Friday. Dr. McCoy told us not to change our plans. I remember thinking *"this must be bad! It will be our last trip for a while."* (Our hotel for our Houston weekend was across the street from M.D. Anderson Medical Center. I told Tom I hoped this wasn't the beginning of things to come.) The biopsy was scheduled for Tuesday, October 6th.

We arrived at the hospital at 6:35 am for my 7:00 am appointment. I was to have a wire put into my breast to guide the surgeon to the lump. Once the wire was inserted we would drive the couple of blocks to the surgery center.

What an ordeal the morning turned out to be! I went to ultrasound first. The pictures weren't very clear so they sent me to mammography to insert the wire while in the mammogram machine. The lump was **too** deep for the doctor to be able to get to it while my breast was being squeezed. One of the reasons they were trying different ways was to go through breast tissue and not my chest cavity. The tumor was deep and sat very close to my chest wall.

I had one nurse that stayed with me and went

everywhere I went, back and forth from ultrasound to mammography. She held my hand and patted it, reassuring me that I had the best doctor doing the wire insertion. Tears started rolling into my ears since I was laying flat on my back. She wiped away my tears and kept patting my arm. The seriousness began to hit me!

When I went to mammography they brought in a second nurse, Diane. I was seated on a stool. One needed to be a contortionist for this procedure! As they placed my breast in the mammogram machine I had to half-stand, half-sit. I was VERY uncomfortable. Diane asked if she could get me anything. I asked, "Is coffee out of the question?" The answer was yes. Instead she rubbed my back. They were taking pictures and were going to use the coordinates, on the film, for the ultrasound doctor to use as he inserted the wires. The other nurse was having the film read to make sure they got the pictures they wanted and needed. Diane continued to rub my back, talking calmly and quietly, as I half-stood, half-sat on the stool with my breast squeezed in the machine. It was probably only 15-20 minutes but it felt much, much longer!!

Back to ultrasound! By this time people were beginning to make comments and patting me as they walked by my wheelchair—not comforting. The guide wires are finally in. I turned my head away because I don't handle medical procedures or blood well. We finally left radiology after 10:00 am to head to the surgery center. I had to get dressed, get in the car, and Tom drove to the surgery center (it was only 1/4 mile but I had to make sure I didn't move the wires). I was starved and ready to have this behind me so I could eat.

Once we were there, they checked my identification then whisked me to the back. They were obviously prepared for me. As I lay down on the table, after changing into the lovely gown (the first of MANY times to come) I remember thinking *"I didn't kiss Tom or tell him I love him."* I just allowed myself to be taken away. It was an unsettling feeling. The next thing I remembered was a nurse asking what I wanted to drink. Nothing.....I wanted to sleep.

Dr. McCoy called at 6:03 the following night. The lump they took out was malignant. I think I knew in my heart it was but to hear the words out loud.....I cried, not sobbing, maybe they were tears of relief. Tom held me and said, "now we know." And that is what we wanted.....to know....benign or malignant. We spent the rest of the evening letting our families know the diagnosis. Mom took it really well. She cried too but I think it was because I was hurting. Janice sobbed... once the initial shock of telling her was over I was okay but she kept crying. Cindy and Kent seemed to take the news matter of factly. I don't know what they did after we got off the phone. Tom talked to his family. And then we waited some more.

I went to see my family doctor. He was the first person, face to face, that I said the words, "I have breast cancer". The compassionate look in <u>his</u> eyes brought tears to mine. I started crying. It was easier to tell people by e-mail or on the phone when I couldn't see their face. Because each person's experience with cancer is different the looks are different—sympathy, compassion, hope, despair, fear, etc. Sometimes I had to be the comforter instead of the comforted!

SURVIVOR TIPS

- Take pencil, paper, and another person with you to appointments. This will help you remember important information.

- Write down questions beforehand so you don't forget when you are sitting face-to-face with the doctor.

- There is hope. Breast cancer is treatable.

Co-survivor in action

When someone tells you they have been diagnosed with cancer, let them talk. Or sit quietly by while they are silent.

Cry with them if that is what's needed.

Don't talk about someone else's bad experience.

Don't talk about your own experience unless the friend specifically asks.

Always remember—every person's cancer journey is different and unique.

My thoughts and feelings:

Chapter 2

EDUCATING YOURSELF

Jean

The medical staff at the St. John's-Whiteside (now St. John's C. H. "Chub" O'Reilly) Cancer Center, in Springfield, MO 40 miles away, was fantastic. One of the first helps was an education class. The education staff invited family/caregivers to attend to learn and understand the same information I would receive. The family/caregivers served as a second set of ears. The education staff helped us know what to expect—side effects; what you could and could not do; dietary restrictions. I received two binders full of information.

Education also happened in the financial area. Family/caregivers were also encouraged to attend this one-on-one session. The financial office searched all insurance plans to find what fit my specific needs best. They were able to find a plan that met all my needs, beyond anything I imagined.

The entire staff was attentive and compassionate towards the patient AND family/caregivers. It wasn't just about the patient. Cancer affects the WHOLE family.

Another help the clinic gave was a *Look Good...Feel Better®* class sponsored by the American Cancer Society. *Look Good...Feel Better®* is a public service program for cancer patients. It is a partnership between the American Cancer Society, the National Cosmetology Association, and the Cosmetic, Toiletry, and Fragrance Association Foundation (www.lookgoodfeelbetter.org). During the session, trained volunteer cosmetologists taught us how to apply make-up, cope with upcoming skin and hair changes and caring for our wig. Then we were given the make-up, donated by cosmetic companies, to "look good." They stressed to us that our lives should be as normal as possible during treatment.

I debated back and forth about going to the class. It was in Springfield and since the death of my husband I didn't do much driving outside of my town. I finally decided I COULD DO THIS and I did! I was glad I participated. The information was helpful and it's always fun to get FREE stuff! Because of this class and wanting to be, look, and feel normal I often had people say to me, "you don't look like you have cancer." To me, that was a good thing. Most people's picture of cancer is a worn-down, washed-out, skinny, hollow-cheeked person. I was not going to be THAT person.

The preliminaries were done. Now the hard part would begin—chemotherapy treatments.

Angelia

Dr. McCoy met with us on October 13 to explain the pathologist's report.

- The lump was 1.5 cm.
- It had clear margins so they were able to get all the cancer.

The next step was to remove some lymph nodes to make sure the cancer had not spread. The surgery was set for October 16th and would include an overnight hospital stay. Radiation is a given and will be done no matter what. Depending on results from the lymph nodes and other tests being run there may be additional treatments. Once lab tests are back and healing is completed, about two weeks, I will be sent to an oncologist and then treatments will begin.

We received more answers but not all the answers yet. Reality began to set in...this is bigger and larger than I thought...It is NOT bigger than my God!

I was very frustrated that we didn't get all the answers I wanted. I like to have a plan and have everything in order and on the calendar. Tell me when, where, and how long this is going to affect my life. The uncertainty of a schedule and time frame was very unsettling for me! It made me very nervous and feeling out of control of my life.

Cindy, the nurse educator, set us up to watch a video about Christus St. Francis Cabrini Cancer Center and what to expect in the coming days. Once the video was finished she sat down and went through a packet of information. The packet contained sheets on my chemo medicines, an emergency room sheet (in case I get sick this lets me by-pass many things in the emergency room), where I can find wigs, their procedures in the treatment room, energy conservation guidelines, foods and medicines to avoid, etc. Of course you have to sign everything to indicate that you understood. I understood at a head level that things would be different, but not how deeply this would affect my life. I signed but I'm not really sure how much I absorbed.

I was STRONGLY urged to be very cautious about being in groups of people because my immune system would be weakened. I also couldn't be around sick people whether they knew they were or not. She also said to discourage hugging. That brought tears to my eyes because I like receiving hugs. I was given a paper to put on my door to warn people about coming to see me if they were sick.

I wanted my mom to be here with me but finding flights on such a short notice (within three days) wasn't cheap. What an impossibility! And where would we get that money? But....our God is good at the impossible and already answered that prayer.

Two friends wanted to provide the funds for mom to fly from Missouri to Louisiana. When I received the e-mail giving me this news I cried. They didn't know what else to do but knew they could do this. The money they sent covered the plane ticket cost exactly!

Lymph node surgery took place on Friday, October 16th. I changed into a beautiful designer hospital gown. This time a beautiful hair cap was added to my ensemble. All the preliminary things were done—any allergies, consent forms to sign, anesthesia, questions to answer. Steve, the hospital chaplain and a member of our church, came in to pray with us. Pastor Bart came for a few minutes, commented on my beautiful hair gear, and prayed with us. Tears welled up in my eyes as I thought, "this is serious."

They took me to radiology to have dye placed in my breast. This was done to determine where the sentinel lymph node was. The dye moves to the first lymph node (sentinel node) that drains close to the cancer site. The dye makes a map pattern of lymphatic fluid. The map can show where the cancer is likely to spread and which lymph node is most likely to have cancer cells. If cancer is found in the sentinel lymph node at the time of surgery, additional lymph nodes will be removed. When I returned from this procedure Kristetta, a friend from church, was in the room with Tom.

They wheeled me through the hallways towards the operating room. Reality once again hit me....this is serious! I've never stayed overnight from a surgery before. The next thing I remember was being wheeled backwards into a hospital room for the night. The most wonderful sight was at the foot of my bed-Tom smiling at me wearing a pink ribbon pin on his shirt!

At some point Angie, the lymphedema specialist, came in and started lifting my arm, changing the way I was laying, giving instructions. I was still struggling to come out of anesthesia and let her do and say whatever she wanted.

I stayed on pain medicine through the night. I got sick once and used the bathroom several times!! I learned quickly that I needed to call the nurse early. I was hooked up to an IV and cuffs on my legs. It took time for the nurses to come to my room and time to get me unhooked.

On Saturday morning a doctor, covering for Dr. McCoy, came in to see me. He looked at everything and said I could go home if I wanted. I wanted to but was I ready? I wasn't fully comprehending everything yet.

Home we went. Tom settled me in. Mable Jo, our next door neighbor, came over to stay with me while Tom went to the airport to pick up Mom. Or at least that is what they tell me. I never saw or heard her. Mom came into my bedroom. I remember saying "Hi" but nothing else.

Mom and I stayed home from church on Sunday. I tired easily. We did go on Wednesday night. People were surprised to see me and kept telling me how great I looked. I'm not sure how I was supposed to look.

I had two drain bottles dangling under my arm. Mom wrote down how much liquid was in each one, detached them, emptied and reattached them. Getting ready in the morning was a long process. The mornings I showered were even longer.

Receiving word that the lymph nodes were CLEAR.... NO CANCER was wonderful!!!! The doctor removed the drain bottles. At that point we knew there would be radiation but we were uncertain about chemo. In my mind that meant no chemo!

OCTOBER 23, 2009

I feel like a cancer patient today. I'm very tired and have some pain. Tom said the drain bottles had loooong tubes inside me. Maybe that is where the pain is coming from. I'll be glad to have the stitches and staples out. Every time I move I'm afraid I will pull them out. Plus I have two holes in my breast! I hope I don't start leaking something.

I'm so glad Mom is here! She's been there. When I say this hurts she is able to tell me if it's normal or not. SHE UNDERSTANDS.

I feel bad having her work in the kitchen, vacuuming,

19

making the bed, helping me shower and dress, etc. But she keeps reminding me that is why she is here.

OCTOBER 27, 2009

Dr. McCoy took out my stitches and staples. He put large tape stitches on. I am to leave them on until they begin to fall off. I still don't look at the incisions much... it makes me weak-kneed and nauseous. I was given appointments for the medical oncologist and radiology oncologist.

NOVEMBER 13, 2009

What a physical and emotional roller coaster the last two weeks have been.

On November 3rd I had to have a PET (positron emission tomography) scan done. I was taken into a little room. A tech came in with big rubber gloves, mask, and other protective gear on and injected a radioactive tracer isotope in my vein. Once he was done they closed the door, turned out the lights and told me to rest for 45 minutes. When those 45 minutes were up they took me to the MRI room where I was placed on a VERY skinny table. The MRI machine was run over my whole body for 25-30 minutes very slowly. This test was done to see if the cancer was anywhere else in my body.

To take the chemo they inserted a port instead of doing a PIC line. By having a port they won't have to look for a vein each week to stick. The port lies just under my skin and allows nurses easy access to insert the chemo.

Port implant surgery took place on November 4th. Some of the nurses recognized me~is that good?! Surgery didn't go as smoothly as expected. I have small veins so they had to make an incision in my neck and go in that way. I was SO cold in the recovery room that my teeth chattered. They gave me Demerol to stop the shivering. As I tried to focus and wake up the nurse lifted my left arm and asked "Did you have this when you came in?" I turned to look at all "four" of my left arms and saw big, red splotches—an allergic reaction. To stop that reaction they gave me Benadryl®. Back to sleep!

Mom said when I came back to the room she couldn't see me—my head was covered in blankets, blankets were piled on top of me. She could see a bloody pillow and that concerned her some. But the doctor explained to her that they had to do my surgery differently. OF COURSE!!

I had my hair cut VERY, VERY short. Hopefully this will make the transition to shaved, then bald easier. We'll see.

I have been so weepy! I am so tired of hurting when I move, not being able to lay on my side, wearing out when I try to do something. And when I think that this could go on for at least a year it is overwhelming. I have to look at it a day at a time. I'm going to be connected to these new doctors in my life for a LONG time. It will be like a marriage. As Dr. McCoy said, "I'll see you till you're 95!"

I thank God for a caring medical team—surgeon, nurses, medical oncologist, radiation oncologist, occupational therapist—even though sometimes they hurt me. These people rejoice in my progress and sympathize and cheer me on during setbacks.

God only wants the best for me. He has provided the best medical staff for me!

NOVEMBER 17, 2009

Another test!

Today I had an ECHO (echocardiogram) to make sure my heart was strong enough to take chemotherapy. It was rather interesting. They place the electrodes on your chest and then run the monitor, with very cold gel on it (I believe I will buy them gel warmers) to take pictures of your heart. Since this was my first one the tech explained what I was seeing. Along with the visual pictures they took audio too. I can't describe how it feels to watch and hear your heart beating.

SURVIVOR TIPS

- Don't be afraid to ask questions. Be an informed patient.

- After a procedure, document aches and pains—anything you are unsure of. Ask your doctor...he/she will tell you if what you are feeling is normal or reason for concern. The only stupid questions are the ones you don't ask.

Co-survivor in action

If your friend has visitor restrictions, make a pretty sign to hang on their door.

Call before going to visit your friend. Once there, limit your visits so you don't wear out the patient.

Provide meals that can be frozen and used as needed.

Make a little port pillow that can be worn under the seat belt to provide a cushion.

My thoughts and feelings:

_____

_____

_____

_____

_____

_____

_____

_____

_____

_____

_____

_____

_____

_____

_____

Chapter 3

THE BIG C—CHEMOTHERAPY

Jean

My cancer was an aggressive type so another surgery was scheduled to remove more tissue to make sure none of the cancer cells slipped out to attack my body in other areas. This surgery took place on the one-year anniversary of my husband's death. A port was inserted to be used for IV chemo treatments. (The original thought was that chemo would be in the form of a pill). The chart, the doctor showed me, shows that this treatment schedule will extend my life by 30 years. I had hoped it would cure my diabetes too!! I never felt the diabetes was a hindrance to cancer. It was probably a help. Because of the diabetes I HAD to eat; otherwise there were times I may not have eaten.

I don't know what I expected in the treatment room. The nurses were super. There was joy, laughter, and hope. From the very beginning there was nothing but hope presented. No doom and gloom. The medical staff worked with me. I was so appreciative that they would do whatever I needed to do, including changing my chemo schedule. Their motto was "make life as normal and happy as possible." At any point, if I had chosen, the treatments—chemo and radiation—could have been stopped.

After my first chemo treatment I felt pretty good. Janice brought me home and her husband, Floyd, was there waiting for us. I went to the kitchen and started preparing a meal. Floyd kept asking me if I felt okay. His only examples of cancer patients had been relatives who'd had cancer many years ago and didn't handle treatments well.

I felt good after the first treatment. I felt more tired after the second treatment. The realization hit me that the chemo was accumulating in my body. This explained why I was tired.

The staff worked with me to schedule chemo treatments to accommodate events I already had planned. In May I traveled to South Carolina to attend my oldest granddaughter's high school graduation. In July I traveled to England to attend the Baptist World Alliance. August brought a trip to Colorado for a short vacation. In September I hosted a cousin's reunion for my nieces. Don't think I was superwoman. There were days when the energy was not there. But God was sufficient. He was so good that He permitted me to teach my adult Sunday School class every Sunday but one.

The chemo treatments were every three weeks and started with a visit with the oncologist. The chemo was customized just for me. Treatments took about two hours—from the Benadryl which kept me from being sick but also made me sleep, to the first chemo, to what they called Kojak juice, which was put in the IV with a syringe. (My son-in-law, Tom, was afraid I'd start craving lollipops and saying, "Who loves you baby?" One of Angelia's co-workers even sent me lollipops.) At the end of each treatment they flushed my port. The last step was to get me awake enough to walk to the car. I felt like gelatin.

When I went in for the third treatment they couldn't access my port for the medicine to flow through. Blood has to come through first or the chemo won't flow properly. It was determined I needed a new port so back to surgery. The new port was metal and I was given a card to carry with me. This only delayed my treatment schedule for one week.

Before each treatment I had lab work done. Chest x-rays, ECHO, and mammograms were done periodically to ensure the chemo wasn't damaging other parts of my body.

I spent Father's Day weekend in the hospital because of severe chest pains. I called my neighbor down the street. We made a flying trip across town to the emergency room. Nancy stayed with me till Janice arrived. The doctor kept me overnight to conduct tests on my heart. All the tests in the hospital cleared my heart but my doctor wanted to be sure! He told me to look at the last possible cancellation date for my trip to England because he wasn't going to let me go until he had answers. I passed the treadmill test and all the pictures with flying colors.

The diagnosis—diaphragm spasms due to STRESS. I told the doctor I really wasn't stressed! I didn't feel it but apparently my body did. The spasms were indirectly caused by the chemo. Chemo made my bones contract which caused the pain.

Chemotherapy kills fast-growing cancer cells. But it can't tell the difference between cancer cells and healthy cells including white and red blood cells. A side effect is low white blood cell counts. It works by killing fast-growing cancer cells. To counteract this I was given Neulasta®. It is a shot, given twenty-four hours after a treatment, to boost white blood cells and reduce the risk of infection.

The trip to England, for the Baptist World Alliance, was a wonderful experience. We attended sessions and I only missed one. We visited points of interest including Stonehenge, William Shakespeare's home, London. Being a tourist meant a lot of walking. Wanda Lee, executive director of Woman's Missionary Union, made sure that I knew it was okay to not attend a meeting or do the activities to keep my energy level up. As a nurse she kept a close eye on me. It was tiring but a dream fulfilled. Someday I will go back and really enjoy England!

One of my husband's nieces commented at his funeral that "it was a shame we don't get together except for funerals." I started thinking and planning and decided all of those cousins (10 girls) needed to spend a weekend together. Because all of them were at least 40+ (in age) the weekend would have a 40s theme. Janice and I collected items, planned meals, Angelia sent out invitations. The big weekend was set for Labor Day 2005.

Everyone came and had the best time. The house was floor to floor girls just like when they went to grandma and grandpa's house (except I have an indoor bathroom)!

We ate, cried, ate, laughed, ate, cried, ate, laughed, ate. Do you see a theme? Sunday morning we took a whole pew at church and Sunday night we had a time of worship around the dining room table (same theme)! It was hard for each girl to leave because it was such a wonderful family retreat.

Wanda, my niece, asked, "How can we pray for you or what can we do for you?" I told her I wanted to help people through this experience. It's not a gloom and doom thing, it's victorious. There is hope.

Life went on during chemo.

Angelia

As a result of wanting my Sunday School class to know how to pray specifically I sent them e-mail updates after each treatment. This was a great way to stay in touch. I also had a group of people literally around the world praying for me.

I was determined that cancer would not change my life. My job was an obesity prevention coordinator for approximately 450 elementary students in a six-parish (county) region. I was also part of the curriculum team that wrote the material emphasizing nutrition and physical activity. Another group of us went into the schools to teach the curriculum to first, second, and third graders. It was a fun job but physically challenging and involved much traveling.

When I was diagnosed my project director, Patrick, told me he would work with me to modify my schedule. I was determined to keep my schedule because that would make me "normal". I soon discovered after each surgery, after the doctor appointments, that I wasn't going to be able to keep that schedule. It was a very high energy job.

Patrick sat down with me and looked at the schedule I had established with the schools. My co-workers, Alicyn and Keli, had already offered to add my schools to their already busy schedules. We decided that I would communicate with the teachers and principals, count out supplies for each classroom and do the paperwork involved. I so appreciated them stepping up and just doing my work even though I thought I could keep up the pace.

OCTOBER 28, 2009

Today I saw Dr. Ule, the medical oncologist, at the Cabrini Cancer Center. After looking at all the risk factors (my age, family history, type of cancer, size of tumor, location of tumor) they felt I should do chemotherapy.

WHAT A SHOCK!!! I knew it was a possibility. None of the others said I wouldn't but they didn't say I would. I was holding out for not doing it. Everything has seemed fairly smooth and easy. So....I thought easy meant no chemo.

As Dr. Ule continued to talk the tears streamed down my face. I think she explained the factors and formulas used to determine how much chemotherapy, what kind, and long but I don't remember any of that. Fortunately she gave me a piece of paper with that information on it. If I do nothing I would probably have a relapse. With hormonal therapy that probability lessens, with chemotherapy it lessens even more and with chemotherapy *and* hormonal therapy it lessens even further. I was thinking about losing my hair instead of concentrating on what she was saying. I remembered how hard it was for me to see my mom the first time without her hair. For me that was the hardest part of her journey and now it would be mine!

I was alone for a little bit after receiving the news. (I had a work meeting so Mom and Tom went on to church.) I just kept thinking about losing my hair. I know that sounds vain but to me that was the worst part of cancer. It is also such a small thing when you consider that this treatment plan will extend my life. I didn't concentrate very well at the meeting. I had other things on my mind and wasn't ready to share this news yet. My coworkers knew about the surgeries and the cancer just not the treatment plan.

OCTOBER 29, 2009

HAPPY BIRTHDAY TO ME!!

It's my 50th birthday. Recuperating from lymph node surgery is not how I thought I would be spending this day. It's a difficult day. I am SO tired and when that happens I can be weepy, and nothing seems good!! It's all overwhelming!

Mom and Tom had a "party" for me. Tom gave me a beautiful pink quartz (birthstone) necklace. It's a good thing there weren't candles on the cake....I don't think I would have had the energy to blow them out. I'm afraid I didn't express my enthusiasm over the necklace very well. Tom kept asking me if I liked it. I do....very much. But when you can barely lift the fork to eat birthday cake enthusiasm is way down on the emotion pole.

As Tom and I lay in bed last night I asked him if it would bother him to sleep with a baldheaded woman.

His reply was, "I sleep with a woman who wears a mask (C-PAP machine). It will be like sleeping with a baldheaded astronaut." My husband, the humorist!

NOVEMBER 13, 2009

I attended the *Look Good...Feel Better®* class at the Cabrini Education Center. *Look Good...Feel Better®* is a public service program for cancer patients. It is a partnership between the American Cancer Society, the National Cosmetology Association, and the Cosmetic, Toiletry, and Fragrance Association Foundation (www. lookgoodfeelbetter.org).

The class had several people just like me! One woman took off her wig and laid it on the table between us. We could be who we were.....women fighting cancer. Each of us was given a bag filled with beauty, skin care, and other goodies from name-brand companies. Local cosmetologists talked about the changes in our hair, skin, and nails, how to cope with the changes and look and feel beautiful. We were also given tips on wearing scarves, hats, or going au natural! I was selected to serve as the make-up model. Anyone walking by heard lots of laughing and probably thought it was a party. It was! It was women forgetting, for two to three hours, they were fighting for their lives.

NOVEMBER 19, 2009

It's been a very LONG day! I started with lab work at

9:30, met with Dr. Ule, then started chemo after lunch. We left there about 5:15.

Here is the treatment plan as of today: once a week chemo for 12 weeks, five to seven weeks of radiation, then back to chemo for once a week to make a year's worth of chemo. So by this time next year I should be finished!!

Once Cindy, the nurse educator, finished with us I picked a recliner in the treatment room. The nurse explained what she was doing as she started accessing my port with a needle. The first thing they gave me was a shot of Benadryl® and an anti-nausea pill. I could feel myself drifting away. The social worker came by to explain the services available to cancer patients. The hospital dietician came by to talk about my diet while I'm on chemo and gave me a list of do's and don'ts. It's a good thing I was sleepy because the food list didn't make me happy.

Then I was hooked up to Cytoxan, Taxotere, and Herceptin®—all with their own set of side effects. The drugs were given one at a time. Each time the nurse hung a new bag she came with gloves and a mask on. It's rather sobering to think they don't want that medicine getting on them and yet they are putting it into my body!

When I was finished I came home and slept! The following day I went back to get a Neulasta® shot, the white blood cell booster to protect against infections.

The Neulasta® shot was not a good experience for me. It was a shot that went in slowly. That wasn't the problem. The problem was the pain I felt afterwards throughout my body. It was a deep, deep ache like nothing I've ever experienced. Nothing seemed to relieve the pain.

NOVEMBER 25, 2009

Heading to the center this morning for lab work (last week's mark just disappeared) and another treatment. Today's treatment is just one medicine—Herceptin®. Next week I will get the threesome. Hopefully just giving me one med and (I think) no white blood cell booster shot I'll have more "energy" days than "no-energy" days this week.

DECEMBER 3, 2009

I started the day at 9:00 am with physical therapy for my arm. Today Tom was taught how to do the therapy to keep the possibility of lymphedema down. Dr. Ule said all of my blood work was good and everything looks good. She seemed surprised to see I still had my hair, but reminded me it could fall out tomorrow! I had a very nice long nap, beginning at 1:00, as I finished up my second full chemo (three meds plus Benadryl® and Tagament). We left the cancer center about 4:30 this afternoon. I usually get to help them close things down.

Tomorrow I go back for my Neulasta shot which is to boost my white blood cell count. It is probably the worst part of this whole treatment process. The ache is deep into my bones. Dr. Ule prescribed pain medication so hopefully it will be better this time around!

I did not follow the instructions given me about my diet and paid dearly! The sheet specifically said "no spicy food". For some reason I didn't think that applied to nachos from Taco Bueno. I was wrong!!

I was just going to eat half but they tasted soooo good that I ate the whole thing. Tom and I headed to the grocery store. About halfway through shopping I started feeling sick to my stomach. I told Tom I was headed to the restroom and I would meet him there when I finished. I used the bathroom and discovered I was bleeding. That scared me!! I must have been in there for a long time because Tom finished the shopping, checked out, and then sent someone in to check on me.

As we headed to the car he asked me if I wanted to go to the emergency room and I told him "let's just go home." Once home, I went straight to the bathroom to sit on the toilet and then I started vomiting. Tom started packing a backpack for the hospital. Then he brought me a lemon-lime soda and a nausea pill. He told me to relax and calm down then we would decide what to do. I'm not sure how long I spent sitting on the toilet bent over a wastebasket. Eventually the pill took affect.

We decided not to go to the hospital. I believe the spicy food and chemo did not mix well. Once I calmed down I felt better, though weak. That episode took what little energy I had left. To this day I have not had nachos from Taco Bueno but I will someday.

DECEMBER 17, 2009

I had my third chemo treatment today. They doubled my treatment today so I can travel to Missouri for Christmas. This means I will skip a treatment next week and my next treatment will be on December 30th. I will receive my booster shot tomorrow. This will only put me one week off but it will be worth it!!

Pray:

- I will feel like traveling by Tuesday—that side effects will be minimal this time.
- No one will be sick in Missouri.
- There is a snow storm expected up there midweek!
- For Tom since he will have to do ALL the driving this time.

This week I was reading on the Susan B. Komen website, www.komen.org, and came across a term that describes those on this journey with us—Co-Survivor. Here is their description *"Thoughtful gestures big and small mean so much to breast cancer survivors, whether they've just been diagnosed or completed treatment years ago. As a co-survivor—because of your strength, love, prayers—you are a treasured source of support and inspiration."*

I had an overwhelming desire to go "home" for the

Christmas holidays. I think I wanted to prove I wasn't sick, I was normal. Plus I felt the family needed to see me, that I was okay. Since our families live so far away (10-15 hours) none of them (except mom) had been to visit.

Tom and I decided we would go to my mom's (in southern Missouri) first since she was the closest (10 hours). We'd celebrate Christmas, let me rest up for a few days, then head to northern Missouri to visit Tom's family.

Everyone, except Cindy and her family, came to Mom's for Christmas celebration. I sat in the wingback chair in one corner of the room. I could see everyone except Janice. We peeked at each other through the Christmas tree.

Who knew that opening Christmas presents was so exhausting! I didn't realize how weak I was. The presents were laid in my lap so they could be opened. One of the gifts was a commercial waffle maker like you see in hotels. I couldn't even scoot it on the floor to take off the wrapping paper.

My brother, Kent, shaved his head. I regret now that my vanity wouldn't allow me to take my wig off and have a bald brother/sister picture taken. That is a moment that can't be recreated.

After the festivities were over and everyone left I realized how exhausted I was. Tom started talking about the possibility of not going further. I didn't want him to miss Christmas with his family so I tried to perk up. I wasn't very good at that! Unbeknownst to me Tom had already talked to his family and told them we may not be coming. Tom, with help from my mom, finally convinced me that it was best for us not to continue to northern Missouri. His family was better with it than I was. Though I was very disappointed I agreed.

I was soaking my hands in water. (A side effect of the chemo was losing fingernails and/or toenails.) When I lifted my hands out of the water they were dark brown. The new color started at the base of my fingers and crawled between my fingers and on my knuckles. The area between my thumb and forefinger was dark too. Tom looked up side effects on the internet and discovered this was one. Later in the evening we noticed the red rash developing on top of the newly colored skin. Since we were leaving the next day to head home we decided to call ahead and go to the cancer center even before we went home!

Cindy, the nurse educator, and Kasey, the physician's assistant, examined my hands and said, "hummm". Not an encouraging sound. The conclusion was that they had never seen anything like this. They took pictures of my hands to put in my medical binder. They were going to keep an eye on this rash. It was finally determined it was probably a reaction to my chemo. Since it was my last BIG chemo they didn't do further tests.

I'm on Week 7 of 12 for the first round. The best news is this was the LAST of the three-med chemo. For the rest of the year I will have weekly one-med treatments. They aren't nearly as intense, just make me sleepy. At this point the five to seven weeks of radiation will probably start in March. I will see the doctor on the 20th and should have more answers or a whole new plan at that point.

I did participate in art therapy today while I waited. It's a program called Cenla Arts & Healthcare. They provide different art experiences in the hospitals and events in the communities. This picture was the hands of different patients. It's an abstract piece. I even got to add my hand to the picture! The woman providing the paints is a cancer survivor and teaches painting at an art gallery in town. I may take up painting!

The red rash on my hands, I started getting during the Christmas holidays, is almost gone. They have decided I had an allergic reaction to something. The rash is turning brown like the rest of my hand (a normal but annoying side effect) and should return to normal in a few weeks.

JANUARY 15, 2010

Made it through the eighth week. From now on I will have weekly Herceptin® treatments, through the rest of the year. We will see the doctor next week before my treatment and should have an update on when radiation will begin. Radiation will be daily for five to seven weeks and as far as I know Herceptin® will not happen during that time.

This past week was probably the lowest for me emotionally. I am weary of treatments. I'm ready to be finished with ALL of this. But as I had plenty of time to think I was reminded of SO many things. These are some of the "lessons I'm learning."

We have two cats, Tac (mom) and Tic (daughter). Tac sees us as a necessity in her life just to feed her and pet her on HER conditions. From the time Tic was young she has followed me around and been my companion. Throughout this journey Tic has been at my side—after each surgery, after each treatment, when I lay down at night. Tic always seems to know when I need to just be able to reach out and pet her, when she just needs to lay close by, when to go off and play, etc. At night she lays at my feet and knows when my head gets cold....she moves to lay by my head to keep it warm. As I move around to get into a comfortable position, she moves away and waits quietly while I get settled, then she moves back in. Sometimes she reaches out with her paw and pats my face as if to reassure me and remind me she is close by.

As I lay thinking (instead of sleeping!) one night I realized Someone else has been doing the same thing. My Heavenly Father is with me through this journey. He is close by, He waits and comforts me even when I don't realize it. He wraps me in His arms to reassure me that He is there and He never leaves me. He knows when my head is cold but more importantly He knows how many hairs will grow back in! He has reminded me over and over that I am His. My strength comes from Him. He knows what is going on and will continue to guide me on this journey.

I am thankful for:

1. A Heavenly Father that loves ME.
2. A wonderful husband who is a fantastic caretaker.
3. For the many friends, family and coworkers— sending notes, praying, filling the gaps at church and work, willingness to take me to treatments, etc.
4. Nurses, doctors, and therapists that act like I'm their only patient and make me laugh.
5. Reminders that my life will be different from now on. I need to be diligent in taking care of this gift God has given me.

As badly as I want things to be the way they were, they never will be. I have a new 'normal". I'm excited and scared about the lessons I'm learning and how God will use these things in my life and hopefully the lives of others.

JANUARY 21, 2010

I am finished with Week 10! All my numbers are good! They are still puzzled by the rash on my hands and thought they may call in experts (which I thought they were!!!). It is something my doctor has never seen before. Compared to the pictures they took of my hands in December, it has diminished some but I will probably have a scar when it is all said and done.

They will be sending me a card for my appointment with the radiation oncologist for February. That will take me into March. Then......it's back to medical oncology to finish out the year with weekly Herceptin® treatments.

Good news—within 6 months my hair should be back to normal. Not as good news—the tiredness and lack of energy can last for a WHOLE year after the treatment is finished. So......in 2012 I'll be NORMAL again! HA!! I am also having problems with lymphedema but that is something I will deal with the rest of my life!

ONE MORE WEEK of Herceptin®!! It was a very quiet day and took a little longer than normal. The computers were down and they couldn't get my lab results. So......they resorted to the "old-fashioned" way...the lab printed out the results and then faxed them to the chemo room.

I did have therapy on my arm today. Lymphedema is an accumulation of fluid when lymph nodes are removed (simple explanation). It causes my arm to swell. When I travel I have to wear a compression sleeve. This is an issue I will have to deal with the rest of my life. I pray that I will be diligent in my exercises, stretching, and elevating my arm but most of all not to get frustrated with this new "normal" in my life.

FEBRUARY 5, 2010

According to my counting I am finished with Phase I! But I have learned that sometimes doctors count differently!!

This week I had an ECHO done on my heart and will have a chest x-ray done next week. This, along with my blood work, will determine if there was any damage done to my body (other than the obvious!). We will see the doctor next week to get the results and hopefully get a date to begin the radiation process (Phase II). Of course I'm sure there will be different kinds of tests to be done for Phase II.

I visited one of my schools this past Monday and taught three classes. I was EXHAUSTED by the time I was finished and a little scared by all the runny noses and hacking coughs I exposed myself to. I had promised to do the other three classes this coming Monday but after that I'm turning it back over to my coworkers. I'll stick with the paperwork!

After five months I think I'm beginning to realize I need to pace myself to participate in activities which means resting up before AND after. I'm also learning that things aren't falling apart just because I'm not there. I don't have to participate in EVERYTHING!

FEBRUARY 11, 2010

Good news:

Started longer every third week Herceptin® treatments today. Tests came back clear which says the chemo hasn't damaged any important organs. I will see the radiation doctor on Tuesday for consultation; Monday (22nd) for my tattoo (radiation markings) and probably radiation the week after that!

Not as Good news:

Blood pressure and weight continue to go up. Will probably have to go on blood pressure medicine but she said once I get my weight down I can probably go off the blood pressure medicine.

Disappointing News:

I thought my food restrictions would be lifted once I went off the BIG chemo but......no. I can't have fresh fruits and vegetables, everything has to be cooked, avoid certain cheeses and spicy food, etc., etc! Do you know how badly I want a salad?!

SURVIVOR TIPS

- If you are given a list of restrictions—food, medicine, etc—adhere to it. Those restrictions are in place for a reason.

- Keep something on your stomach to avoid the nausea. Because mom (Jean) is a diabetic she was required to eat six times a day. I (Angelia) lived on different kinds of crackers, white soda, and hard candy for several weeks. People will tell you different things to help with nausea. Try them and choose what works best for YOU.

- Find a breast cancer survivor support group through your community, church, or hospital. Participate in one that is upbeat. It's good to share stories with someone like you but don't let it drag you down. You don't need to be discouraged during this pause in your life.

- Find a *Look Good...Feel Better®* class near you and participate. Take a friend with you. Playing with the make-up and scarves is fun!

Co-survivor in action

Prepare meals for the family for an extended time. The cancer journey is a long process. Space them out so the family is not overwhelmed with food. Ask about food restrictions—the patient may or may not have restrictions.

Provide restaurant gift cards.

Pick the children up from school. Take them to their after-school activities.

Mow the lawn or shovel the snow.

Plant flowers or work in the garden.

My thoughts and feelings:

_____

_____

_____

_____

_____

_____

_____

_____

_____

_____

_____

_____

_____

_____

Chapter 4

WHERE DID I PUT MY WIG?

Losing your hair can be an emotional and traumatic experience. In my case (Angelia) I lost hair everywhere—head, legs, eyebrows, eyelashes, underarms. I didn't completely lose my eyebrows and eyelashes. Mom lost ALL of her hair—no eyebrows, no eyelashes, etc. And to this day she still doesn't have to shave her legs.

A friend and I were discussing this recently. Rhonda said, "The hair loss is really an identifier that one is a cancer patient. When it starts to come back a part of your identity is gone. Even though it's a devastating loss it is still an identifier. You want people to know that you didn't CHOOSE to cut your hair this short!"

Jean

Since chemo would probably make me lose my hair the oncology nurse suggested I have my head shaved so I wouldn't have to experience the trauma of my hair falling out in clumps and my head getting sore. I contacted my hairdresser for an appointment. She was so gracious. Peggy offered to come to the house but I had her schedule an appointment at her salon. I wanted to feel normal and not "sick". I was scheduled as the last customer of the day. She was finishing with a customer when I arrived for my "hair" appointment. While she was waiting on the customer's hair to finish drying, she washed my hair. Peggy explained later that others didn't need to know what was about to happen. Washing the hair was "normal". Once the customer left Peggy locked the door and drew the blinds. She turned me away from the mirror. While she was shaving my head I thought, "this is another step in the process that HAS to be done. This is one of the times I realized "I have cancer....this is real." If I pretended before I can't now. The scars are hidden but hair loss isn't. It is outward and always there as a reminder. Then....hair gone. Peggy placed the wig on my head, hugged me, and sent me home. My first look in the mirror at home was shock. My head was so white!

My daughter, Janice, would rub my head and say, "You have such a sweet round little head." My son, Kent, shaved his head to empathize and support me. Later I lost my eyebrows and eyelashes. I actually didn't realize I had lost them till Janice mentioned it one day. I knew my face looked different in the mirror but I hadn't pinpointed the reason.

The American Cancer Society provided wigs free of charge and had an area set up at the cancer center. There were a variety of styles, colors, and lengths. My first wig made me look like an old woman, even though I am one. That wig was later exchanged for another, more becoming, for which I got many compliments. I also wore turbans around the house. As time progressed I was more comfortable in not wearing anything on my head....but only in the house.

The hair came back in almost overnight. I went to bed one night bald and when I got up the next morning someone had planted a garden of black stickers on my head. They were prickly and very black. I had never had black hair. It was difficult to sleep because of the prickly feeling hair. As my hair got longer it laid down better. It wasn't long before one could tell I had hair again.

The first hairs around my face were very curly and black. As it grew it became straighter and grayer. My hair returned to its original state except it is a little bit finer.

Angelia

Losing my hair is the most difficult thing I may or may not be facing. Mom sent me scarves and turbans and I bought a couple of scarves that can be used afterwards. I've been practicing tying them. I will use them because I was told that you lose heat through your head and since it's colder out I need to keep my head covered even at night. Tom said jokingly "as normal as you are, you will probably lose your hair after the last chemo treatment".

Tom and I picked out a wig before my hair began falling out. I wanted to have one on standby and not have to go through that choosing process as I was losing my hair. The wig shop called to say my wig was ready but I chose not to pick it up until I needed it.

Dr. Ule was very surprised that after my second chemo treatment I still had hair. She told me I might be in the small percentage that doesn't lose my hair. I prayed that was true!

DECEMBER 7, 2009

Had a bad hair day.....as in it started falling out. I went in to take my shower, put shampoo on my head, started rubbing it in and big chunks of hair came out. I stood in the shower and SOBBED!!! I beat on the shower wall as I cried out. I collected myself and rubbed my head again to make sure this was really happening. It was happening. I sat down on the shower floor, screaming and crying.

When I dried my hair more came out on the towel. I e-mailed Tom that IT (losing my hair) had started and we'd have to pick up my wig after work. I would make an appointment to get my head shaved. Of course this happened on a Monday when most hair salons are closed.

My wonderful husband came home, when he received my e-mail, to hug me and tell me I would be his favorite bald person. I had composed myself from the earlier shower incident. When Tom wrapped his arms around me the tears started flowing again. After lunch we went to the shop to pick up the wig I had ordered several days earlier (and hoped I wouldn't need). We went from there to the beauty parlor to have the wig styled and my head shaved.

Tom suggested we see if the salon at JCPenney's was open. I had met Melissa, the manager, at a *Look Good, Feel Better®* class before this. We walked in and I asked for Melissa. When she saw me she knew why I was there. She hugged me, my tears started again, and she took me to a private area in the back. She styled the wig on my head and then gave me a mirror to see how I liked it. Melissa took the mirror away and began to shave my head. I wanted to look but knew I would start crying again. Hearing the buzz of the shaver reminded me this wasn't an ordinary hair cut. What a wonderful Christian woman God sent! We talked about our churches and our faith.

It took me several days before I could look in the mirror and not cry. My wig hung on the doorknob just outside of the shower. When I stepped out of the shower I immediately put the wig on my head.

I had my meltdown and probably will again until I get use to this new look. But I know the God who knows how many hairs I have and need!! One Scripture keeps running through my mind. Luke 12:7 says, "Indeed, the very hairs of your head are all numbered. Don't be afraid; you are worth more than many sparrows." (New International Version, NIV)

I do have 5-10 longer hairs that are standing straight up on top of my head. I'm not sure if they are white or blonde but I'm going with blonde!! I don't think my hair will come in as fast as it went out!!

DECEMBER 2009

I'm becoming more comfortable with not wearing my wig around the house. Usually when I come in I take it off and throw it on the back of the couch. That way if someone comes to the door I can just grab it and throw it on before answering the door. I'm not comfortable with other people seeing me.

JANUARY 2010

I went shopping for a new outfit. Of course, every time I pulled something over my head the wig shifted. So....I would take it off, put on the outfit, then put the wig back on and show Tom the outfit. Once I came out of the dressing room and Tom kept motioning with his head. He wouldn't say anything, just kept moving his head. Finally he said, "You forgot your wig." I guess I'm more comfortable with my bald head than I thought.

MARCH 5, 2010

On the hair side—I may have to buy my first bottle of shampoo since last September! It's beginning to thicken a little. Not enough to go without covering in public (according to me)! I do have some longer straggling strands too.

MARCH 25, 2010

In the hair department I can now hold some strands of hair, on my head, between my fingers. It's pretty dark so far. Instead of standing straight up and feeling prickly it's beginning to lay flat and feel soft. I also got to shave my legs this week (never thought I'd be excited about that!!)

APRIL 9, 2010

On the hair front—I have 3-4 hairs that I can pull behind my ears! YEAH!!! Maybe in a couple of weeks I'll feel comfortable enough to go without my wig.

APRIL 29, 2010

HAIR UPDATE: The unveiling will be May 1st!! The wig is coming OFF! It's beginning to get sweaty when I wear it. If you are interested in a wig (slightly used!) let me know!!

MAY 23, 2010

Tom has started call me "Curly". My hair is still thickening up and very curly. When I get hot it REALLY curls! We'll see how much curl stays as it gets longer. I am thankful I don't have to wear a wig in this heat and humidity.

SURVIVOR TIPS

- Once your hair starts coming back, begin using a shampoo/conditioner for damaged hair. Your hair texture, color, straight/curly may be totally different after chemo.

- I (Angelia) had my hair cut very, very short before I started losing it. It helped the transition somewhat.

- Celebrate not having to shave your legs!

Co-survivor in action

Let the patient grieve over their hair loss—tears, anger, etc.

Buy or make bright, colorful scarves, hats, or turbans.

If your friend normally wears earrings buy large dangly ones.

Encourage your friend to be daring with her wig choices.

My thoughts and feelings:

_____

_____

_____

_____

_____

_____

_____

_____

_____

_____

_____

_____

_____

_____

_____

Chapter 5

RADIATION AND THE TATTOOS

Jean

Before radiation I had a cat scan so the tattoos could be placed on my body. Tape was placed on my body to know where to put the tattoos. The tattoos were small ink dots where the radiation would be focused. Three weeks after the chemo, radiation treatments began for six and a half weeks, Monday through Friday. Every few days I met with the radiologist.

The hardest part of this treatment was laying completely still. I was afraid I'd mess it up because I have a hard time laying still. I had a coughing fit. It was no problem for them. They just waited till I finished coughing. The last week and a half the radiation was more focused and intense.

People from my church made a schedule to transport me to the radiation center in Springfield every day. The driving part of the trip took two hours. This made the radiation treatment even more tiring. They waited patiently during the fifteen minute treatment. It bothered me that people had to travel two hours for that short appointment. But it never bothered them. Often they insisted on taking me to lunch after the treatment. Some even bought an extra meal for me to take home to eat at dinner time. That was going above and beyond! These lovely people had servant hearts. They were truly Jesus with skin on.

My hair started coming back during this time. I was excited about the dark and wavy hair but it didn't stay that way. It quickly became straight and white. My eyebrows and eyelashes were back now too.

Angelia

My first appointment with the radiation oncologist, Dr. Menache, was painful. I didn't have full range of motion with my arm. That didn't stop them from doing x-rays and examining my breast and underarm area. After the exam it was decided I was a good candidate for MammoSite. This way of radiation involves inserting a balloon catheter into the lumpectomy cavity. A radiation "seed" is delivered through the catheter attached to the balloon. I would receive two doses—one in the morning and one in the afternoon—for five days. This sounded so much better than six weeks of radiation. Once I was finished with that I saw the medical oncologist. Dr. Menache said to me that day, "The first day you wake up after your diagnosis, you are a survivor." I have heard him say it many more times to many people.

We went shopping in preparation for radiation treatments. I needed some tops that were loose-fitting, easy to get on and off. Mom and I also shopped for a lounging outfit that I could wear between each day's treatments. Something comfortable but that covered me well if someone dropped by for a visit. Sports bras, with front closures were also on the shopping list. We found some cute things. I also found some no-rinse shampoo. Showering was out of the question so this was an easy solution to washing my hair. These were my "radiation clothes and tools".

When Tom and I started this cancer journey I got a little frustrated that we didn't have all of the answers and timelines when I wanted them. After the first two surgeon appointments I realized it's better to get a little bit of information at a time and have a chance to absorb and process that bit of information before going to the next appointment. On October 28th (the day before my birthday) I received overwhelming news that took time to process—Chemotherapy will be a part of my treatment plan. Right now radiation will go as planned in November and a couple of weeks after it is completed the chemo will start.

I went back to see Dr. McCoy to have the balloon inserted for the one-week radiation. They sent Tom out of the room. The company representative (for the radiation balloon catheter) was in the room with us. The needle was inserted into the lumpectomy incision and was very tender. Dr. McCoy was trying to insert the needle and use an ultrasound machine to determine where the cavity was located. Though he numbed the area I could still feel the digging movement......not good! Dr. McCoy kept saying "mmm" "mmm" "mmmm" and it didn't sound like a good "mmmm". They decided to try to put a saline solution in the cavity to see if they could expand it.

WHAT PAIN!!!!!! He stuck that needle in and moved it around. That is when I wanted to say, no scream, 'no MORE!!!' I don't remember the last time I hurt that bad. The company rep suggested a longer needle but thankfully Dr. McCoy said no.

The good news is I heal fast. The cavity, where the radiation balloon was to be inserted, is almost closed up—less than 1 cm. The bad news is I will have to do radiation the old-fashioned way. Instead of twice a day radiation treatments for a week I will do several weeks of daily radiation. I went ahead and kept my appointment with the radiation oncologist to go to Plan B. I was very disappointed. This didn't fit into my plans to get this all over with and move on with my life. Plus I had "radiation clothes and tools!" But then I was reminded of Isaiah 55:8—"For my thoughts are not your thoughts, neither are **your** ways MY ways," declares the Lord (NIV). Yes Lord!! Knowing that in my heart didn't keep my head from trying to analyze why this happened this way. The treatment plan was changed. I began chemotherapy the following week.

I have been so weepy! I am SO tired of hurting when I move, not being able to lay on my side, wearing out when I try to do something. And when I think that this could go on for at least a year it is overwhelming. I have to look at it a day at a time. I'm going to be connected to these doctors for a LONG time. As Dr. McCoy told me, "I'll see you till you're 95!"

I have had several people tell me how painful radiation is. They said it was so bad they stopped taking it in the middle of the plan. I was DETERMINED that I would see this through to the end. I am trusting my doctors and my God that they know what is best for me. I can't imagine not doing the treatment if it is going to kill the cancer cells and/or prevent them from returning!

FEBRUARY 16, 2010

We are back from the radiation oncologist. Today was an informational meeting. On the 22nd I will go back for an examination and to have markings (tattoo) put on my skin.

Radiation begins on March 1st and will continue for six weeks and three days. (Not sure why they don't tack on two days and make it seven weeks! Tom says by the end of the six weeks and three days I will be glad they didn't add the two extra days.) According to my calculations I will be finished with radiation on April 14th. I will have three chemo (Herceptin®) treatments during the process also.

The main side effect is the possibility of skin irritations. I have very sensitive skin (bandages leave rashes) so my prayer is that my skin will toughen up for the next couple of months!

FEBRUARY 22, 2010

I now have black and blue "tattoos". There are 10-13 "cross" markings with tape over each one—three down the middle of my chest, one above the affected breast, one on the breast, one under the affected breast, three down my side by the affected breast and three down the opposite side. These markings help them line up the laser. I was told there are no side effects or restrictions..... except

- I may have skin reactions and irritations (knowing me probably!)
- I can only use a certain deodorant, no lotions or creams on the radiated areas, only 100% cornstarch instead of powder, only 100% aloe vera for irritation.
- I may get tired towards the end of the treatment.
- No water aerobics because we're not sure how the chlorine will react to the radiation or markings (probably erase them).

Other than that, (and any others that I may discover!) I'm good to go and should have no problems. HA!

My first treatment is Monday at 11:30. I will also have a chemo treatment that week, meet with my medical oncologist, and meet with my family doctor about my blood pressure. It will be a busy week!

MARCH 1, 2010

I had my appointment in radiology today. I had more markings added and more x-rays done. At least they didn't add another color!

Actual radiation will begin tomorrow at 1:30. It will take place every Monday-Friday at 1:30 till April 15th. I pray that my super sensitive skin will be toughened to handle this treatment.

MARCH 2, 2010

Grandma Brown died today. We knew she was very sick. She had asked Tom years ago to preach at her funeral. Unfortunately I'm not going to be able to go. This makes me mad! I want to be with the rest of the family grieving with them. I don't want to be home by myself. I want to support Tom as he preaches her funeral and grieves for her. I didn't even get to take Tom to the airport! I had ANOTHER doctor's appointment. I'm so tired of these interrupting my life. I want NORMAL!!!

I made it through the radiation part okay. As I was sitting waiting to see Dr. Menache tears started rolling down my cheeks. Janet, his nurse, asked me if I was okay. I told her Tom's grandma had died, he had gone to Missouri, and I wasn't able to go. I was having my own little pity party. She was comforting. She told me if there was anything they could do while he was gone to let her know.

Once I had my pity party I felt a little better. I really didn't want to have my pity party in front of Tom. He felt bad leaving me but I would have felt worse if he had been here with me and unable to honor his grandmother's wishes. My job, right now, is to take care of myself. The rest of the world will have to take care of themselves without me.

They called me in for my radiation treatment. They gave me a "lovely" gown and showed me a locker to place my clothes. Then I went behind the BIG doors for my treatment. I laid on a table with my arms up over my head holding on to pegs while they moved a machine around me. My instructions were to lay still and breathe normally. When I'm told to breathe normally I feel my breathing is restricted. I get short of breath. Is my breathing really normal? I shouldn't think about it.....just do it.

I was also told to let them move me when they made adjustments....don't help them. Do you know how difficult that is? Since there was just a "Go Saints" poster on the ceiling I started thinking. Doesn't God tell us all the time to let Him do the work? He is in control.

Just let Him make the adjustments. We don't have to do anything. We don't have to help God; He can do it!! It brings to mind Jeremiah 29:11-13, "For I know the plans I have for you," declares the LORD, "plans to prosper you and not to harm you, plans to give you hope and a future. Then you will call upon me and come and pray to me, and I will listen to you. You will seek me and find me when you seek me with all your heart." (NIV) Why do I have to be reminded? Why can't I just relax and let God handle it?

MARCH 5, 2010

By 2:00 this afternoon I will be finished with day 4 of 33 treatments. It has been a difficult, long, tiring week—beginning this phase of treatments, Tom's grandma dying and him leaving (he'll be home day after tomorrow—YEAH!!), family doctor appointments, etc.

Yesterday as I lay on the radiation table I thought I can't do 30 more days of this; I don't WANT to do 30 more days! I wondered what would happen if I told them I was finished. I dismissed that thought from my mind quickly. Especially since I have the routine down and they don't have to tell me each step. Besides they did all the work of setting up the computer and marking me so I'd hate to throw all of that away. The other thought that struck me was, "God must have a LOT to say to me. I'm on this table for the next 30 days...silent and laying perfectly still." So... when I got home yesterday afternoon I decided I'll go

back today, the day after, the day after, the day after....
until ALL 33 treatments are done.

Now about the radiation table...it could be a carnival
ride. It goes up and down, forward and backwards, side
to side AND they can make the top half move from the
bottom half. I must have a crooked body because they
have to move the top half to get the laser lines to line up
with the markings on my body. OR maybe the markings
are crooked.

I thought I would feel the laser but I only see those
red lines in the air going through my body. I guess I'll see
the effects of the laser beams.

I did meet with my medical oncologist yesterday and
will NOT be doing the Herceptin® with radiation. That is
a relief! I won't go back to see her for about seven weeks
which means no more lab work for a while.

I will meet with the radiation oncologist every week
and have x-rays done every week. Since I've started
treatments I've added almost 20 pounds. This week I had
lost a pound which I was excited about. The doctor told
me I couldn't lose any weight during radiation. (Have you
ever had a doctor tell you that?!) My prayer over the next
few weeks is that I won't gain any more and I'll TRY not
to lose any more.

As I went into radiation Friday the nurse said to me,
"I always see you with a smile on your face, whether
it's in the waiting room, treatment room, or wherever."
It was an answer to prayer. When this journey started

for Tom and I we wanted God to be glorified in ALL of it...whatever that entailed. I've tried to be real. It's not easy being sick but it's not always easy being a Christian either. BUT there is joy in all of it.

The radiation countdown continues! Even though the routine seems to stay the same there are slight changes. I had x-rays done to see how the treatment was going. They connected my black, blue, and green lines with purple lines (I'm quite colorful now!) Once they drew the lines they took photos for my notebook. I am a very well-documented person! Add to this the fact that my skin is beginning to pinken. The doctor says that is okay as long as it doesn't go red!

Tom and I are fighting colds. Thankfully we are feeling better. The hardest part was finding a medicine I could take. I have a whole page of things I CAN'T take. Today I decided I was probably going to survive this cold.

MARCH 18, 2010

Today was day 13 of 33 radiation treatments. Dr. Menache is in New York so I had a substitute doctor—a woman with a Scottish brogue. She was in and out so I didn't get to hear her talk as much as I would have liked. She did tell me that I looked the way I should at this point in the treatment—which is like a slight sunburn. The nurse told me that from this point on I will probably lose my appetite and my energy. We'll see.....I gained weight during chemo because I was HUNGRY all the time! I even made supper tonight for the first time in several months. Hopefully there will be more of those events.

My head is getting darker which means my hair is beginning to come back in. There are a few long stranglers but mainly the hairs are short. I wonder why it doesn't come in as fast as it goes out?! Hopefully by summer I can be rid of the wig because it is not very cool.

Tic, the younger cat, woke me early this morning eager to get her day started. She followed me closely as I began my morning routine. She didn't seem to want breakfast or to go out. She was content just to be with me...sit by me, cuddle with me, be in the same room. It is sad that sometimes I don't have that desire to be with God. To be in the same room with Him and spend time with Him. That is my prayer for this week—to have the same desire, and act on it, to be with God that Tic has to be with me.

MARCH 25, 2010

Another week of radiation almost done—YEAH! I will have a reprieve on Good Friday. Everything is good. I have to use aloe vera and hydrocortisone cream as needed. I also found out today that I will get to ring the bell at the cancer center when I finish radiation. It is quite a ceremony.

This week has not been that great in the "feeling well" department. I've decided I don't like cancer! I know it's a little late but I guess I'm a little slow. The fatigue has been overwhelming and frustrating. I apologize to anyone (especially my caretaker Tom) for being whiny this week. But this too shall pass!

I find myself spending more time outside. Some of it is because that is where Tom spends so much of his time. Some of it might be because spring is more precious this year. I've enjoyed watching the new life. The green pushing up through the brown earth. The yellow, purple, red, orange, pink flowers that pop out. And that's just the FLOWERS. It doesn't count the green onions, cabbage, lettuce, tomatoes, green beans, mustard greens and peppers growing.

Feeling the breeze. Watching the clouds float by. Laughing at the cats playing in the yard. Amazed as they sit by me as I rock and contemplate.

APRIL 2, 2010

Radiation reprieve!! I finished day 23 of 33 yesterday and the cancer center is closed today so I have three whole days without a medical appointment. AND I have a distinct hairline! Celebration day!

Another treatment yesterday, another marking added. They added a circle around the scar where the tumor was removed. My last five treatments will be focused and more intensified in that spot. Right now I'm looking a little bit like Neapolitan ice cream with blueberries. Some of my skin has darkened (chocolate)

73

which I also experienced with chemo. Some of my skin is white (vanilla) where the radiation doesn't touch. Other parts of my skin are pink (strawberry) where the radiation hits. Surrounding all of that are the blue markings (blueberries)!

I listened to the heavy doors shut as the radiation techs left the room yesterday to give me the treatments. The realization struck me at the magnitude of what was happening to my body. I began to wonder if I had asked enough questions, is it too late to ask questions, etc. But these people have been trained and I'm not the first person they have treated. I can trust them with my treatment plan.

So.....am I that trusting with God? Sometimes not! I ask questions, I whine about why, I sometimes question His wisdom. Shouldn't I trust Him more than anyone? YES! He knows and wants what is best for me. This Easter weekend I want to remember the magnitude of what Jesus did for ME.....He died for my sins so I wouldn't have to. More importantly He was raised on the third day and lives in me today, right now, tomorrow, and forever. I will spend eternity with Him. Who better to trust my life and plans with? "For I know the plans I have for you," declares the LORD, "plans to prosper you and not to harm you, plans to give you hope and a future. Then you will call upon me and come and pray to me, and I will listen to you. You will seek me and find me when you seek me with all your heart." Jeremiah 29:11-13 (NIV)

APRIL 9, 2010

I am FINISHED with week five of radiation. And a good thing too...my skin is beginning to react to the tape. It could be a combination of the marker and the tape! This means I can wash and scrub off all the markings except the circle around my scar. Week six will be focused, more intense and concentrated levels in the tumor scar area. They will put an extension on the radiation machine that gets right down to my skin. Hopefully it won't feel any different from the past five weeks.

I've probably felt more discomfort this week than the past few. There is a noticeable change in the look of my skin. On the plus side the techs and nurse told me I'm "normal". Not a word used often in my medical history!

I have coined a new term—fatirex. It means "beyond fatigue, beyond tired, beyond exhausted". The fatirex hits me suddenly and I have to lay down and sleep. So frustrating!! Someone told me this week they could tell I wasn't myself, I looked/acted like a puddle. I think that was a good description. I was a puddle that didn't move until someone stepped in me; then I could ripple along and move ever so slowly to the next spot and wait for the next step to ripple me on.

It's hard to believe Phase II is almost finished. At times it seemed like the treatment was dragging. And other times it has moved quite quickly. I am thankful again that I live so close to the cancer center. This treatment only disrupts part of my day and then I can resume life. For others that must travel this journey, it has taken a chunk out of their lives.

APRIL 16, 2010

> It is finished, the battle is over
> It is finished, there'll be no more war
> It is finished, the end of the conflict
> It is finished and Jesus is Lord.

Words and music by Bill & Gloria Gaither

This song has been playing in my mind the last few hours. I still have more traveling on this cancer journey but.....the radiation phase is FINISHED. A few tears were shed....of joy! I really can't describe right now what I feel. I told Tom as we walked out of the cancer center, "maybe life can go back to normal....whatever that is. I feel like the past six weeks my life has been put on hold and revolved around that 1:30 radiation appointment."

I will still be monitored closely for the next 18 months by Dr. Menache (radiation oncologist) and my skin has to heal. But.....I'M DONE WITH RADIATION!!!! Now on to Phase III (which I think is the last as far as treatment goes). I will see Dr. Ule (medical oncologist) on the 29th and will go back on Herceptin® for a while.

They took the remaining tape off my skin. I was surprised to see white skin. Obviously the radiation didn't go through the tape. I am very colorful. My radiation techs, Chris & Anne, made a potentially uncomfortable situation comfortable. It must have been....I got used to taking my arms out of the hospital gown and laying bare-breasted on the table.

I have had days filled with frustration. Replies to my e-mails and Facebook posts talk about how strong and brave I am. Not all the time! I am frustrated by:

my lack of energy—I can't do the simplest things without resting;

not being able to eat a salad—I think I'll only eat salads when this is over;

not traveling—this is the longest I've been "grounded";

not being able to do things with Tom—I like going with him even if I don't enjoy the activity;

not feeling like exercising—I can't start water aerobics (maybe) until after my May 18th appointment with Dr. Menache;

the blisters under my breast, right where my bra sits, and the soreness of my lymph node scar.

SURVIVOR TIPS

- Nursing pads worn under your bra will keep your bra from rubbing raw radiation skin.

- An aloe vera plant relieves the burning. (Be sure to check with your doctor that this is okay. He/she may have restrictions while you undergo radiation.)

Co-survivor in action

Provide rides to and from treatment.

Provide meals for the family.

Do the laundry.

Clean the bathrooms.

Provide taxi services for the family.

Take care of the car—wash, oil change, etc.

Do the grocery shopping.

My thoughts and feelings:

Chapter 6

BACK FOR MORE CHEMO

Jean

After radiation an additional treatment was begun, Herceptin®. This therapy specifically targets tumor cells that overexpress the HER2 (Human Epidermal growth factor Receptor 2) protein. This treatment does not increase chemotherapy-induced side effects. It would be every three weeks for a year. Herceptin® was to lessen the possibility of the return of the cancer. It was administered by IV as the chemo had been. In my case, I finished chemo, I finished radiation, and then I started the Herceptin®.

While on the Herceptin® treatments I was asked to participate in the American Cancer Society's Relay for Life. The Relay For Life is a community event that gives everyone a chance to celebrate survivors and remember those who didn't survive. It is a 24-hour event and teams have a representative walking at all times raising money for a cancer cure.

The Laclede County Relay for Life is held at a local park. I went to walk the Survivor's Lap and was amazed at the number of survivors of all ages—men, women, AND children. At the Survivor's Tent we were given a T-shirt and a pin which I wear proudly. As we took the lap I was humbled. When the announcement was made that the survivor lap was starting, people flocked to the path from every point in the park. They stood on both sides of the path cheering and clapping. The cheering is more about the act of survival than the individual. Survivors are set apart as a model that cancer can be beat! I began to cry like a baby because I was so touched. I continue to participate. What an encouragement this experience has been and is. You realize you are a SURVIVOR!

When the Herceptin® was finished I was given a cancer prevention pill as a part of a clinical trial for post-menopausal cancer patients. If you heard shouts coming from southwest Missouri on November 16, 2006 it was not an earthquake. It was shouts of hallelujah and thanksgiving because I finished chemo! It was a long 1½ years! but God was so good to me and my family through this process. Not only were we dealing with the ups and downs of cancer but we were still deep in grief over losing husband and father. But God was faithful on this journey. This trip would have been too hard without Him.

Angelia

APRIL 29, 2010

After almost two weeks without doctor appointments (except the eye doctor and ENT) I saw my medical oncologist today. I'm looking good! I am leaving bits and pieces of my radiation skin peeling all around.

Phase III with Herceptin® only (15 treatments) began today. As Dr. Ule explained it, Herceptin® is a chemo with antibodies. It does not have the same kind of side effects normally associated with chemo. So....what little hair I have will be staying. According to her I will be done with this treatment in January 2011. According to my calendar 15 treatments end in March but I'm sticking with her timeline!

Phase IV with Tamoxifen also began today. It is an every day pill that I will take until April 2015! It is used to treat patients with early stage breast cancer. It can also be used to help prevent the original breast cancer from returning and prevent the development of new cancers in the other breast. It has its own side effects. I hope I can keep all of these side effects straight!! If I understood her right this pill prevents my estrogen from attaching to any possible cancer cells and spreading. For the treatment of breast cancer this medicine greatly outweighs the risks!

I'm beginning to regain some energy back. I hope to do some traveling over the next couple of weeks for work. Traveling tires me....I can get to places but sometimes getting back is too much! I don't travel by myself right now.

MAY 23, 2010

I finished another treatment on Thursday and saw my radiation oncologist this week. All restrictions have been lifted for my skin—I can start water aerobics again, wear any kind of deodorant, wear powder, etc. All my blood counts, platelets, heart, kidney and lungs are good! They are pleased which makes me pleased!!

I am on an every third week chemo schedule which means......the other two and a half weeks I can be "normal". I visited classrooms for the last time during the school year (with the help of drivers). This week mom has been visiting and we've actually done a few fun things.

It's hard to describe the feeling of being so close to the end of treatment....only eight more months! I feel like I'm beginning to get my life back. The previous eight months are a blur which could be a good thing. Pacing myself to not use up all of my energy is difficult. I try to cram a lot into those two and a half weeks before chemo.

JUNE 10, 2010

I finished another treatment today. Obviously my numbers were good or they wouldn't have given me the treatment. We switched things up today and sat in a different place! I think we confused the nurses. I also had my first mammogram this week since my diagnosis. I'm going with "no news is good news"! I'm seeing the effects of chemo on my nails now. It was explained to me as "just like my hair quit growing so did my nails. They have begun growing again and the ridge lines are the indicators of growth". At least they didn't fall off! They tear easily so I have to keep them cut short.

I began going back to water aerobics last week. It felt good to be in the water! I only lasted 30 minutes but it is a start. I look forward to building up my stamina again.

I've been looking forward to the "every third week chemo" schedule. I'm ready for life to be *normal* again. Then I thought maybe I better look at the definition of normal. And here it is.....normal as defined by Merriam-Webster Dictionary is: **a.** according with, constituting, or not deviating from a norm, rule, or principle **b.** conforming to a type, standard, or regular pattern.[1]

I determined I have three different kinds of *normal*— bc (before cancer), dc (during cancer and treatments) and ac (after cancer and treatments)!

BC Normal—I did everything everyone else did— went to church, work, travel, play, water aerobics, ate what I wanted, etc.

DC Normal—going places has been limited to staying out of crowds; eating has been limited to eating processed and cooked foods (nothing raw or fresh);

---

1   Merriam-Webster Dictionary

traveling has been limited because it is VERY tiring; my skin is different; my hair was nonexistent and is now different; naps are a part of my daily routine; lymphedema is a constant battle and something I have to be diligent about; continuous testing to make sure the medicines aren't messing with my body; Tic, the cat, has been a constant companion (she must sense I'm getting better because she doesn't hang as close....though it could be she prefers being outside in the warmth); exercise wears me out but I'm beginning to build up my stamina, etc. My *normal* is different.

AC Normal—looking forward to this time! I can eat salad!! Tom and I are planning a dinner out and I'm going to have the BIGGEST salad ever! I will have to be more diligent about taking care of my body with diet, exercise and monitoring.

The ONE constant through this whole journey has been my Heavenly Father. He has not changed and has walked beside me and carried me when I couldn't walk. I pray that my relationship with Him isn't *normal* anymore. I feel more of a burden for people than I have ever known before. This is something I don't want to change-I want it to become a new *normal* for me.

My life is definitely going to be different from now on....it began changing with the diagnosis in October 2009. I pray that it is a good difference....one that will make a difference in someone else's life. I don't know what lies ahead but I know WHO knows and is already preparing me for that. I don't know if God will change my ministry focus or just change me and how I minister to others. That journey continues......................

So many people have told me "how good I look". I believe that is good. Some days I have to work at it because I don't really feel as good as you think I look!!! Make-up is a wonderful invention.

JULY 26, 2010

After my June treatment we went to the Carpenter reunion. We decided I could sleep in the car just as easily as at home! When we arrived my mother-in-law had injured her knee so she and I kicked back in the recliners with our legs up and got a lot of visiting done! Because of my sun restrictions I spent most of my time in the house and had a lot of one-on-one time with Grandma Carpenter (who turns 95 in August!) I pray my mind will be as sharp when I'm that age; but it's not starting out that sharp so we'll see! It was good to see everyone.

I had another treatment this past Thursday (22nd). All of my blood work is good AND I had lost three pounds. Unfortunately business is up at the cancer center so the staff was hopping. In a couple of weeks I will be seeing my medical oncologist and my radiation oncologist and then more tests! It's all a part of my progress report!!

I AM WEARY!! I have nothing—no desire, no energy, no want to—NOTHING! I can't remember the last time I have felt so desolate, so empty. Maybe I'm tired of being strong. I just want to curl up someplace, alone, until everything is right again. I think there are several things that are contributing-not spending enough time with God and in Scripture, heat, wondering if my job will be funded after August 31st, laziness, low energy, ongoing ear problems, etc. I have really struggled the last few weeks of being weary of all of this. Then I am reminded:

1. There are more treatments DONE than there are left to do.
2. I have an incredible support system.
3. God ALWAYS provides ALL of our needs.
4. There is a reason.
5. There are others who have MORE to deal with than I do.
6. I have hair!.....and everyone tells me how cute my curly hair is.

So.......I'm going to put on my big girl panties. God and I will conquer this. He is SO much bigger than any of this. It's in His arms that I need to rest.

AUGUST 9, 2010

I was reading 1 Corinthians 13 today. Even though I have read this Scripture many, many times before what stood out this time was that love trusts and protects. I saw Tom in my mind as I read that Scripture. He has taken care of me and protected me always but even more so over the past few months. I thank God for him. I'm not sure how I would have handled this without Tom by my side.

AUGUST 10, 2010

I see the end getting closer but sometimes it seems to drag!! I get a little discouraged when others diagnosed after me are already finished with treatments. It somehow doesn't seem fair! My heart is full of SO many things but my mind is totally blank.

AUGUST 13, 2010

I saw the doctor before my treatment yesterday. All of my numbers were good except blood pressure and weight (which are probably related!). Tom mentioned to her that I get short of breathe. She listened to my heart and lungs a little bit longer. She thinks it could be related to the extra weight but to be on the safe side she has moved my heart ECHO to be done next week. One of my medicines has a side affect of causing heart trouble. Today I'm feeling a lot like I did after some of my first chemo treatments. Hopefully it's a combination of things and I'm not regressing!

I will see the radiation doctor next week for a follow-up visit. We are still on target to finish chemo in January; then there will be a BIG party....with salad!!!!

FROM LIMBO TO DISCOURAGEMENT TO ACCEPTANCE (not all the way there yet): When I got home yesterday afternoon I found out that the appeal to fund our jobs was turned down. Needless to say, it was a shock and I was very disappointed. I have worked in this program for eight years and worked with some great people. We are in the process of closing out the project and I will officially be unemployed after August 31st.

This week I have talked with God about all of this several times. I picked up a devotional book written by a good friend that she gave me a few years ago. The Scripture, commentary, and questions this whole week have been about letting God handle all the details (or at least that is what I gleaned from it though that may not have been the author's intent). The following is from that book. This commentary is related to John 2:8-10 and the miracle at the wedding at Cana.

"Mary was quietly confident the matter was safe in His hands no matter what He decided to do. Jesus chose to perform this miracle perhaps to teach us that no matter how attentive to details, we may be, our best cannot begin to compare to His. He may have performed this miracle to remind us that we needn't worry when we're "in a pinch." He is more than capable of getting us out. He may be reminding us today that He is much more interested in our hearts than He is with our hands."[2]

I was praying that the "miracle" to be performed would be keeping my job. Obviously that wasn't it. Now I wait for God's "miracle" in meeting our needs. Of course

---

2   *Women Touched By Jesus* by Leighann McCoy

I have already given Him my list but I will wait and see what He gives me. I'll be honest there are still moments of tears, why?, doubts, etc.....But deep in my heart I KNOW He will take care of us. He always has and I have seen that so much in the past few months.

I pray that my heart is in line with His and that I will be confident in the way He chooses to show Himself. Which means......I have to quit taking it back and figuring it out.

AUGUST 15, 2010

I think I've regressed after this treatment! I DO NOT feel good! achy, and cold, in 100+ temperatures. I've even slept with the blanket on at night! VERY unusual for me. Tom thinks I might have picked up a bug at the hospital. It does have many sick people.

AUGUST 16, 2010

Today begins the journey of building back up my energy. I stayed home from church yesterday. I think I would have been fine but just the thought of driving tires me! Will this feeling ever leave? To see something that needs to be done and just get up and do it. To not think through how much of a task I can complete before I'm worn out. Do I need to push myself or let my body dictate what and how much I do?

AUGUST 20, 2010

My appointment with Dr. Menache was good. He said my numbers were good, my liver was functioning, and my blood pressure was down a little bit from last week. AND my June mammogram came back clear! I am very thankful we have insurance to take care of our medical expenses. I can't imagine having the financial stress along with the physical and emotional stress right now.

SEPTEMBER 1, 2010

I think I'll begin counting down how many treatments I have left. It gives me a goal! I feel I've lost a year sometimes but I've gained so much encouragement and support from others! We are so blessed! I read this Scripture today—"The earth is the Lord's, and everything in it, the world and all who live in it. Who is he, this King of glory? The Lord Almighty—he is the King of glory." Psalm 24:1, 10 (NIV)

SEPTEMBER 13, 2010

Another full week without doctor appointments.... soon this will be the normal. That day is getting closer and closer. Whatever shall I do?

What a year it has been! Would I have skipped it? Yes and no! God has worked in my life in ways that would NOT have happened if it weren't for this journey. He continues the work He started. I am a different person because of this journey, hopefully, a better person. It hasn't been the easiest journey but the company (people) who have journeyed with me have been amazing!

Thank you God for ALL the people You have placed

in my life "for such a time as this." The new friends, the family, the continued friendship of others.

This kind of sounds like good-bye. In some ways it is. Good-bye to a "sick" life and hello to what lies ahead.

SEPTEMBER 24, 2010

I had chemo last Thursday. Instead of counting how many months I have left (January sounds so far away!) I've decided to count how many treatments I have left. *Drumroll............*There are EIGHT (8) left!!! YEAH! Hopefully they will continue to go as smoothly as they have been. Of course I still have the doctors who want me to grace them with my presence over the next few months. The "tube in my ear" surgery went well. At my follow-up I was told I didn't have to come back for another six months.

The past couple of weeks haven't been the greatest. My last day of work was August 31st which is also the day Tom's truck died. My computer died on Thursday. Of course I complained to God as if He didn't already know what was going on in our lives. One of the devotions I read this week in *Women Touched By Jesus* reminded me that we need to ask for what we really want. Sometimes, because our faith is small, we misjudge the character of God. We ask for what we think He wants to hear from us. It's not like He doesn't know what is in our hearts. SO.....this week I have been specific about the kind of job I want knowing that He will provide all of our needs.

I know He only wants what is best for us. Is it easy? No, not always. But there is a peace that can't be explained except that I know Who holds our future!!

Keep February open because there will be a BIG PARTY with salad and fresh fruits and vegetables to celebrate!!!

SEPTEMBER 29, 2010

We've been attending a Financial Peace University class at our church. After this week's class it clicked! Even though I have lost my job we can live on Tom's salary by budgeting. We have to be diligent and make some sacrifices but it is doable! This will relieve some of the pressure and stress I feel to find a job. Now I can focus on treatments and regaining my energy.

I was watching Tic this morning. She's sitting at the bottom of the fence, looking up as if she is trying to figure out the best way to get to the top. She looks to her left but rejects whatever she saw over there. Suddenly she gets very still, her ears perk up and she LEAPS! She is on top of the fence, all senses on alert. She is very intent on whatever she is after (probably a bird). I have no doubt she'll succeed.

How often do we sit and look up at the insurmountable task ahead. God is there with His outstretched hand saying, "LEAP, you can trust Me!" I only have to take the hand and He will guide me through.....whatever the seemingly insurmountable task.

OCTOBER 6, 2010

Another treatment finished! I have only six left! My blood work was good—liver & kidneys functioning, oxygen, blood pressure lower. I will have another heart ECHO done in November. I think they gave me a double dose of Benadryl® though. I slept hard during treatment, came home and slept, slept last night AND still feel like I'm in a fog.

January looks far away, but when I look back over the past year, January looks much closer! I'm thankful for a "fairly easy" journey….especially when I see others at the Cancer Center who seem to be having a more difficult time. I have hair, I am back at water aerobics, I can travel with Tom when he goes to preach out of town (though I do get tired!), I have my piano students back, I do a little cooking, some ironing. Life is good, though I do get frustrated with my low energy.

October is Breast Cancer Awareness Month. Make sure you get a mammogram!!!! A mammogram detected my tumor early and saved my life.

OCTOBER 7, 2010

"I will refresh the weary and satisfy the faint."-Jeremiah 31:25 (NIV)

"He heals the brokenhearted and binds up their wounds." Psalm 147:3 (NIV)

This time last year I was preparing for a life-changing

experience. I can't believe the many different people who have touched my life AND the many people's lives God has allowed me to touch. WHAT A JOURNEY!

One year ago today I heard the dreaded words, "the lump was malignant, it is cancer" and thus began the journey of learning. I was suspicious when I saw the lump on the routine mammogram several weeks before. It was good to have an answer and now our lives could proceed.

What a journey this has been! If I had the choice I would not have had this experience. As I look back on the past year there are SO many things to be thankful for:

- my husband who threw our healthy eating lifestyle out the window and stocked up on snacks that had previously been banned from our pantry, so that something would taste good; and for being my rock.
- the nurse that saw it was close to time for my yearly mammogram, called the doctor to get orders changed and the lump was found on the side that we weren't going to test.
- doctors and nurses, phlebotomists, radiation techs, front desk people, pink ladies (the hospital volunteers who provide blankets, drinks, bring your lunch) that show compassion when they are telling you the facts; who cry with you when your hair begins to fall out; who

rejoice with you when the wisps of hair start peeking out under the wig, who celebrate the baby steps.

- co-workers that stepped in when I just knew I could carry my load and be superwoman while undergoing chemo and radiation treatments.
- family that called, sent notes, cried with me, helped me recover from surgery, touched my fuzzy head, shaved their head (you don't know how much that meant to me Kent)!
- for my church family that sent virtual hugs when I had to limit my contact with people; who took me to chemo to watch me sleep and didn't laugh at my drug-induced stupor.
- for new and old friends around the world (literally) who have prayed and encouraged from afar.

This journey <u>has</u> been a blessing! I can't describe the peace that I have had—even on the very few "today I feel like a cancer patient" and "today I'm mad that cancer is interfering in my life" days. I have had a hard time saying "I had breast cancer" My radiation oncologist says, "the day after diagnosis you become a survivor!"

SO.......I AM A BREAST CANCER SURVIVOR!!!!

Though I still have six treatments (4 months) left, in this leg of the journey, I am changed forever. I can't wait to see what God has in store for us now....to use what I'm learning on this journey........in the days ahead.

OCTOBER 25, 2010

What a week and a half it has been! In case you've been hibernating October is Breast Cancer Awareness month and I've been able to participate in some activities.

Sunday, October 10th, was the 10th Annual THREADS, a fundraiser for Cabrini Cancer Center's patient assistance fund, at Alexandria Riverfront Center. This fashion show honors local cancer survivors. All the proceeds stay in Alexandria to help Cabrini patients with transportation, medicine, meals, supplies, and other costs during treatments (Fortunately Tom and I haven't had to tap into this fund but it is very helpful for others—especially patients that come from a distance).

I was privileged, along with 79 other cancer survivors, to be a model. What an experience to see so many cancer survivors and their co-survivors. My husband, in-laws, and coworkers represented some of my co-survivors.

My in-laws left on Thursday as Tom took me to chemo. My numbers were good (my blood pressure is finally settling down!!) and I enjoyed my nap. I can't believe I'm so close to the end. YEAH!!! November will be filled with more tests to make sure my organs are still normal (and no they don't do any tests on my brain so don't even ask about that test!) and two chemo treatments.

On Saturday, October 16th, Alexandria had their first Susan G. Komen Race for the Cure. I did not participate but went to watch many friends who did participate. Words cannot describe the emotions as I watched 4,000 people run/walk that 5K. Soooo many people walking in honor and memory of people they know and love who have been affected by breast cancer. The cheers, the tears, the laughter, the somberness of the disease... it was a very emotional experience. I have made the commitment to do the walk next year. It will be on Saturday, October 15, 2011. Come join me!!

It was good to be reminded that I'm not alone. There are many people affected by this disease....some more so than others. I have people surrounding me with love and encouragement—my husband, my family, my church family, my friends and coworkers and One who has never left my side.

Needless to say I'm going to rest the remainder of the week. Thank you again for your prayers and encouragement.

NOVEMBER 8, 2010

We are now down to FOUR treatments left!!! The end of January is getting closer!

The blood work was good, the blood pressure was high, the heart test was good, the weight was down! Some side effects have raised their little heads so will be going to regular doctors to get baseline information and make sure they don't cause REAL problems.

It's hard to believe that this day is finally coming! This time last year it seemed like it would never come. Though I have a treatment on Thanksgiving Eve this Thanksgiving I will remember the love of my Father; the support and encouragement of my husband, of family, of friends. There is SO much to be thankful for.....even in difficult and trying times.

NOVEMBER 28, 2010

I had a treatment on Thanksgiving Eve. Numbers were good, I've lost two pounds and the countdown continues! I also saw the surgeon this past week. After my last treatment in January the surgery to remove my port will be in February. And then it will be over......except for follow-ups!

This Thanksgiving season has been a time of reflection....remembering where we were this time last year and being thankful for so many things:

1. Hair—last year I had none; this year I have LOTS of unmanageable curls!
2. Family—so very thankful for my wonderful husband, mom, siblings, in-laws, cousins, aunts and uncles
3. Church family—what wonderful encouragers and pray-ers they have been
4. Friends—rides to the doctor, notes, prayers
5. Our Father's provision—even though I have

been out of work since September all of our financial needs have been met

6. My health—yes, I've had cancer; yes, I've had some rough days but those have been outnumbered by the good days; yes, I'll be tethered to my doctors for a long time but I can handle that; there are others that are having a harder time than me with their cancer treatments.

7. My medical team—what a cheerful group of people who always make it seem like I'm the only patient (I have noticed they do that with others too!)

Now I look forward anxiously to the end of treatments. It will come quickly but the anticipation and waiting seem far, far away. I sometimes feel like that little girl that waited for that first snow day. We watched the snow fall the night before. I'd listen for mom to go to the kitchen, she'd listen to the radio. If she didn't holler down 'breakfast was ready' or 'time to get up' I knew I could snuggle down in the warmth of my bed and enjoy my snow day! So........I will snuggle into the comfort of my home, family and friends as I anxiously await the day the doctor says "You are finished!" and I get to ring the bell.

And now on to Christmas! Take time during this season to reflect on the most precious Gift!

DECEMBER 3, 2010

Central Louisiana lost a beloved one on Wednesday-Coach Janice Joseph-Richard (ree-shard). I didn't really know her except through the Pink Ribbon Club (breast cancer support group at Cabrini Cancer Center). She always smiled and had an encouraging word.

She served as co-chair of the Susan G. Komen race this year. Her third relapse of cancer seemed to shrink her little by little. Her treatment schedule was about the same as mine.

Coach Richard had a treatment on Thanksgiving Eve. Someone wheeled her in. She smiled and said "Hi!" as she rolled by my recliner. I told Tom she looked very tired and weak. Her friend was wheeling her into one of the treatment rooms.....reserved for those who need to receive treatment in a bed.

Before she went into the room she stopped by the chair of someone receiving treatment. She asked her how she was doing, smiled, and laughed. I don't know if she knew the person or not. I'm not sure it mattered.

I don't know why her death has affected me. I didn't "KNOW" her. We were nodding acquaintances at best. I was more of an observer of her life.

I am saddened by her death. She lost her five-year battle with cancer. And yet she is a Christian so she is HEALED and celebrating!

Are there people observing me as I receive treatment,

attend meetings, do errands? Will their lives be happier, encouraged because they have seen me?

Maybe that is why her death has affected me. It has given me pause to reflect. Father, let my life make a difference to others around me.

"When my heart isoverwhelmed, lead me to the rock that is higher than I." Psalm 61:2 (NIV)

DECEMBER 16, 2010

I had a treatment yesterday and saw Kasey, the nurse practitioner. The weight hadn't changed from last time (*good that I hadn't gained any, bad that I hadn't lost any!*); blood pressure still a little high but all other numbers good!

The light I have been seeing at the end of the tunnel may be a small train instead of open sunshine! When I mentioned that I was excited to have only two treatments left in January there was a pause as she looked through my thick medical binder. "You're on #13 and we usually do 17 treatments. It's possible to only do 15...we'll see." I'll probably find out for sure in six weeks which is when I see the doctor next. SO........I may not be done till March 10th instead of the January 26th **I had planned**!

Yesterday's treatment was a little rough. When I finished Suzanne, the nurse, asked if I felt okay. Tom said I didn't look well. She wanted to get me a wheelchair to meet Tom but I walked.....verrrry slooooooowly to the front door. I slept for five hours when I got home and went to bed early last night. Tic came in when we got home, waited for me to settle into bed, then crawled in beside me! Today I still feel a little achy and sluggish.... more so than normal!

Last night Tic and Tac tried to lay with me on the couch. Tac would distract Tic (*I think Tic is ADD because it doesn't take much*) and jump up into her spot. Then Tic would do something to cause Tac to run after her! They finally both found a spot beside me that they were happy with.

I wondered......does my Father try to get my attention like that......especially this time of year? I'm distracted by so many things around me—cleaning the house, finishing Christmas presents, sending Christmas cards, worry about a job and finances, etc. I've heard SO many saying how much they have to do—shopping, baking, decorating, etc. Let's not get distracted by the glitter and lights. Remember that the first Christmas was very rustic and simple! There wasn't much fanfare....just the animals, parents, shepherds and the angels. Don't forget WHY we celebrate Christmas....the coming of the Babe.... so we can celebrate Easter!

Sit down and read the story of His birth and take time to celebrate!! Have a MERRY CHRISTMAS! I can't wait to see what 2011 will be!

JANUARY 11, 2011

Happy New Year to each of you. I pray God will guide and bless you through this new year.

We enjoyed our visit to Missouri. We left, from Merryville, LA on the 27th and returned in time for my treatment on the 6th. Saw a little bit of snow, lots of cold, lots of food, and most of our family members.

Treatment went well. I had gained six pounds (YUCK!!!!!!!!!—I think it was fluid from being on the road for two days—that's my story and I'm sticking to it!); blood pressure was a little better than it has been; lab work numbers good. Because of some issues/side effects I'll be having some tests run. I was told this isn't out of the ordinary though.

The chemo nurse told me my last treatment will be January 27th. I see the doctor that day so I will wait to hear her say those words. Excited but apprehensive! Many, many thoughts running through my mind that I will try to organize and share at another time.

JANUARY 28, 2011

Yesterday morning I got up with excitement..... anticipating my last chemo treatment. I'll admit I even dressed up a little (a nice top and make-up!) so I would look good in the picture of me ringing the bell to signify the end of my treatment!! AND.......it didn't happen. **I have one more treatment on February 17th.** I knew there was the possibility but on this journey being optimistic helps.

My numbers look good and the doctor seemed very pleased. I will be going to Shreveport to do genetic testing to see if I carry a breast cancer gene and for any other kind of cancer. No....we don't have children but this will benefit my siblings, nieces and nephew.

Yesterday was a very long day! Unfortunately all the chairs were full and the whole process took longer! Our neighbor, Dian, came in during her lunch hour for her chemo treatment. She said to me "you are my role model and my hero." I've thought about those words and what she meant (I was under the influence at the time!). I decided to look up the definitions. According to the *American Heritage Dictionary*, role model means *'a person who serves as a model in a particular behavioral or social role for another person to emulate'* and hero means *'a person noted for feats of courage or nobility of purpose, especially one who has risked or sacrificed his or her life.'*[3]

I don't feel like a hero! and I'm not sure how good of a role model I've been. It does serve as a reminder that people are watching us and everything we do—how we handle a grumpy cashier, how we handle standing in a long line, how we handle ourselves in traffic, our countenance in the waiting room, etc. I guess Dian has seen me handle myself well on this journey but more importantly how has my Father seen me handle it? I want to be the role model and hero that people will say, "there is something different about her and I want

---

3   American Heritage Dictionary

that too!" What kind of role model and hero are you to those around you?

SURVIVOR TIPS

- Set small goals for yourself.
- Don't be discouraged by what is still ahead; celebrate and rejoice in how far you have come.

Co-survivor in action

Send an encouraging note or uplifting card.

Send a plant or fresh flowers.

Provide gift cards to the family's favorite restaurant.

My thoughts and feelings:

_____

_____

_____

_____

_____

_____

_____

_____

_____

_____

_____

_____

_____

Chapter 7

HALLELUJAH DAY!

Jean

December 6, 2006 was Hallelujah day. On that day the port was removed in the doctor's office in a matter of minutes. I was thankful that everything went well because the next morning I was scheduled to teach the International Mission Study at my church. Now I felt the treatments were completely over. I now wear the purple ribbon of a breast cancer survivor proudly! Even though treatments are finished I will be monitored closely by all oncologists and on a cancer prevention pill for the rest of my life.

Once the clinical trial was finished, at my one-year, ALL CLEAR appointment, my oncologist sent me for genetic testing. Because of family history they wanted to know if I carried a cancer that would be passed to my children. The genetic testing of the BRCA1 and BRCA2 genes, included washing my mouth out with mouthwash and spitting in a cup, three times. I then added my saliva to the cup. Once the results were back they would give them to me and discuss my options for further cancer prevention treatments. The results were negative. No gene mutations were found.

Then.....three and a half years after I finished MY treatments the news came that my daughter, Angelia, had breast cancer. And another journey began. This time the news was more disturbing than when I was diagnosed-she was my child. But I knew there was hope because of all the new treatments constantly coming. More than that, God was in charge.

Angelia

FEBRUARY 17, 2011

IT IS FINISHED!

No more chemo! Yesterday was my last chemo treatment.

My lab numbers were good...perfect were her exact words. I did show her both of my big toenails which are now a different color. She looked at them, said "mmmmm.....this is normal for Herceptin® but it usually doesn't happen this late in the treatment." Again I choose to be different! I am having some issues with tightness and swelling in my arm (lymphedema). If it continues I will go back to the therapist. But….lymphedema is an issue I will deal with the rest of my life.

I didn't get to ring the bell! My treatment was finished during the lunch hour and my doctor wasn't there. They gave me the option of waiting for her or ringing at another time. Since I have an appointment with my radiation oncologist on Tuesday I'm going to go a little early and ring it then. Besides….there was only one person in the lobby. When I ring it I want the lobby to be FULL! I want everyone to know I'M FINISHED!!!!!

I shed a few tears and sat, almost in shock, after they took out my IV. It's been a long journey…..not a horrible one…..but one that I pray won't be repeated! I feel like our lives have been on pause for the past 18 months. It's hard to express in words my emotions right now. There seems to be a whole new world out there. Have my priorities changed? I pray so. Am I different? I think so. Will I do things differently, see people differently? Yes. Will I monitor my health closer and encourage others to do the same? YES! Will I miss my Thursday afternoon long naps? Yes….but not the Friday draggy feeling!

What's next?

1. I now start my three-month check ups; then six months, then yearly.
2. I will be going to Shreveport to participate in a genetic study.

3. I see the surgeon on March 3rd to schedule the port removal.
4. The house will get a THOROUGH cleaning..... that might take awhile. (I've been told it could take up to a year for my energy levels to return.)
5. Learn to manage my curly hair!
6. I'm going to spend a week with mom.
7. Look out world, here I come!!

Salad bar, here I come.....soon!

FEBRUARY 22, 2011

Upon reflection I have decided there are four steps to finishing chemo. I have now completed three of the four! Yeah me!!

The four steps are:

1. Finish the actual chemo.
2. Ring the bell!
3. Eat foods from my restricted list which are now unrestricted.
4. Have my port removed.

I rang the bell today, February 22, to signify the end of my treatment. My medical oncologist wasn't there again. I was given the choice to go ahead or wait till a day she was there. I chose to go ahead. It's just one step closer to being done and I'm ready to be done! My radiation oncologist is the one who did the announcement. The others who celebrated with me were my chemo nurses, nurses, and physician's assistant. They do celebrate with you! as if you are the only person they are treating. What a special group of people!

Salad, or anything fresh or unpasturized was on the restricted food list. Tonight we went to Applebee's. I ordered an Oriental Chicken Salad. I was expecting the half-size but got the full-size. I enjoyed every last bite!! There is a whole new world of food opening for me.

I will see the surgeon on March 3rd to set the date to have my port removed. On March 17th I go to Shreveport for the genetic testing. As long as there are milestones I will celebrate!

MARCH 15, 2011

I will be having my port taken out at 9:30 this morning. The doctor says it's a simple procedure. I'm praying that is true....I don't always do things simply.

On Thursday we go to the cancer center in Shreveport for genetic testing. THEN I think I will be done with doctors until I start my three-month checkups.

MARCH 17, 2011

Tom and I went to Shreveport for genetics testing and counseling. I had to fill out a questionnaire ahead of time and mail it back to them. This meant contacting cousins to get information on aunts and uncles. I put X's in the boxes for every family member with cancer. Two or more X's means a person is predisposed to developing cancer. I had six X's.

The hereditary cancer educator charted my family cancer tree. The test I was having done was a comprehensive BRCA1 and BRCA1 Gene Analysis. According to clinical data from Myriad Genetic Laboratories I had a 40.7% chance of a mutation. Carriers of this mutation have a 50% chance of developing breast cancer by age 50 and an 87% chance by age 70. There are also higher risks for a second breast cancer and ovarian cancer. These are sobering statistics. Because of our family history I wanted to arm my three siblings and five nieces and nephew with all the information.

My blood was drawn. We went home to await the results.

APRIL 7, 2011

I just got back from Shreveport and getting the results from my genetic tests. I'M NORMAL!!!! (keep your comments to yourself)

There was no mutation on the breast cancer genes. I think the educator was very surprised given my family history. This means my risk for developing breast and/or ovarian cancer is lowered significantly. It could be from other hereditary genes but not the BRCA1 and BRCA2. At this point I go back to my oncologist and hear her recommendations (which will probably be the normal monitoring) and continue my life. My next appointment is May 3rd. I think I get to see ALL of my doctors and surgeons in May!!

I'm now ready for a nap. A friend went with me but I did the driving-four hours round trip. It's the longest distance I have driven in a LONG time.

SURVIVOR TIPS

- CELEBRATE! It has been a long journey and you have finished it!

- Keep up with follow-up appointments and testing.

- Share your story. You don't know who needs to hear about your journey.

Co-survivor in action

Celebrate with your friend/family member.

My thoughts and feelings:

Chapter 8

BECAUSE OF THE JOURNEY

Jean

As I look back over the past five and half years I'm still amazed at the peace that was always present. That only comes from God. I don't ever remember being angry about the illness but I did wonder why it happened when Lonney wasn't there to be my support system. I learned so much—patience, allowing people to minister to me, listening to what God wanted to teach me, using my experience to minister to others and the kindness and compassion doctors, nurses and other staff showed.

There were so many supporters during this time: family—they will never know how much they meant to me—love was in abundance. Kent, my son, shaved his head in support of me losing my hair. He helped change my insurance as suggested by the financial advisor from the cancer center. I never knew what Thoma Sue, my niece, would be sending. Once it was an afghan, once it was a candle, a portable CD player. I never knew when or what would arrive at my door but it was something I needed that particular day to lift my spirits.

Cindy and Angelia, my daughters, came to visit when they could get off work and took me to treatments. Neither one of them could watch as the nurses accessed my port. Cindy couldn't watch during the treatment. She brought a book to read and sat with her back to me. Janice took me to the rest of my chemo treatments. She laughed with and at me when I was goofy with medication. She was an encourager through the journey.

My church family was tremendous, always doing helpful things and praying. They brought food, visited, took me places just to get out of the house. The WMU family prayed and encouraged through notes and e-mails. A support system makes a great difference in encouraging a cancer patient. One Sunday School class member told me frequently "you don't look like you have cancer." I'm glad.....you see I knew God was making me look normal. When you are going through cancer it becomes your total focus. Letting people in helps you not to be consumed by medicines, doctor visits, and treatments. If you become self-centered during your journey it is not beneficial to the healing process. There is hope. If you decide there isn't, you might as well give up.

Philippians 4:7 became my verse for this journey "and

the peace of God, which transcends all understanding, will guard your hearts and your minds in Christ Jesus". NIV

Receiving notes and cards at the 'right' times was such an encouragement. God knew when I needed them. It was a blessing to receive them and know I wasn't on this journey by myself. Everywhere I turned there were people to help. It was like there was a whole army to walk beside me.

The Ladies' Auxiliary, at the cancer center, made port pillows. These were 4" x 6" stuffed with cotton batting. I kept it in the car to put between my port and the seat belt as a cushion. Baskets always set in the chemo room with the port pillows and turbans in them. These were for chemo patients to take as needed.

I give God ALL the glory for His presence, His strength and His guidance. Without Him the journey would be impossible. The song that runs through my mind is

"Through it all, through it all,
I've learned to trust in Jesus, I've learned To trust In God.
Through it all, through it all,
I've learned to depend upon His word."

By Andrae' Crouch

Angelia

As Tom and I began this cancer journey our prayer was that whatever happened God would get the credit and glory for it. We wanted people to know Who is taking care of us.

CaringBridge website—If you have friends and family spread out across the world having a website is a great way to keep in touch and let them be a part of your journey. Mom and I didn't use one but we have had several friends that have used them. Go to http://www.caringbridge.org to set one up.

Let people help you—When people offer to do something for you LET THEM! They wouldn't have offered if they weren't willing and don't let them miss out on the opportunity to minister to you. As I looked back at e-mails, I had an offer for housecleaning. I did not take her up on that because my house was messy and I thought it would have to be cleaned before she came! I appreciated Kristetta as my driver. She rode with me to my schools. I could get there fine but by the time I was ready to come home after teaching classes I would be too tired to drive. Kristetta, Liz, and Mable Jo drove me to chemo treatments when Tom was unable to.

Second set of ears—You always need a second set of ears when you go to the doctor. If a family member can't go with you ask a trusted friend. As you are listening to the doctor, especially at first, there is so much information that is thrown at you. You need someone to listen <u>with</u> you. Write it down!

Side effects—there are side effects and risks involved. Be aware of them but DON'T dwell on them. If you dwell on them you will be focusing on the cancer and the medicine and not on getting better. Beating cancer is 80% attitude and 20% medical.

I developed a rash on my hands. They also turned dark down between my fingers and on my knuckles. The doctors weren't sure what caused it....more than likely an allergic reaction to the chemo. They took pictures from all angles and added it to my medical binder. I was told it would probably leave a scar (discoloration). I decided I would use it as a reminder to pray for others who are on this same journey. The rash eventually disappeared.

Humor—Finding humor in the little things is a tremendous help. My husband was a great help in finding humor in things. He bantered with the nurses in the chemo room. He helped me to laugh. Tom, most of the time, knew when not to laugh.

Be honest with your doctors—If you have a pain, ANY changes, tell them. It may or may not be related to your cancer or the treatment. After being fussed at for not telling them I had tremendous pain for two-three days after my Nuelasta® shot I learned to tell them everything. They were able to give me a low-dose pain pill. This allowed me to go back to my "normal" routine quicker. Nothing is too small. The doctors are the ones with the medical degree and years of experience. They will make the determination if it's serious or normal. Most of my complaints were considered normal. At first, I wondered why they didn't alert me to different side effects or pain.

I soon realized they deal with so many patients with different kinds of cancers with different kinds of needs and other health issues. They can't remember to tell us everything. I may not have the same issues as someone else.

Radiation issues—I did have problems with skin reaction to the radiation treatments. Not every one does. I still have some blistering, a year after finishing radiation treatments, and now use aloe vera and my husband's handkerchiefs tucked under my bra.

How others saw my journey—Shortly before this journey began I had been convinced that as Christians we need to be specific in our prayers. When I started sharing through e-mails, with my Sunday School class, I was very specific in what I wanted them to pray for. I tried to be very open with them—sharing the good and the bad days!

Five months after my diagnosis, Steve was diagnosed with leukemia. It was difficult news to hear. I guess in the back of my mind I thought no one else would ever be diagnosed with cancer again. At least not anyone I knew! Because of his low immune system he was confined to home and people weren't allowed to visit. Denny, his friend, came to me at church one Sunday and told me how upset he'd been when told he couldn't even go visit his friend. Then he remembered an e-mail I had sent about a weakened and compromised immune system and understood better. He told me "thank you for those e-mails....it helps know how to better minister to Steve." That was our (mine and Tom's) purpose and prayer all along.

Listen to your body—As humans, especially women, we don't always listen to what our bodies are saying. We are so desperate to not look or act "sick" that we overcompensate. If you add stubbornness to the equation it is not good. It took my boss, Patrick, driving four hours to my house and sitting down with me saying, "you don't NEED to do this schedule." (My work involved writing curriculum and then teaching the lessons about physical activity and nutrition to first, second, and third graders in a six-parish region. I was on the road a lot!) He didn't tell me I couldn't do my work; I didn't <u>need</u> to....my health was more important. Alicyn and Keli, my coworkers, divided my schedule and added it to theirs. I made the arrangements, pulled the supplies together, and did the paperwork and reports.

It took my husband asking why I thought something needed done before I understood he was protecting me and my health. I didn't need to be superwoman. I could still keep my schedule somewhat but I needed to add rest time before and after.

Take your time getting back into your routine after treatments. Your body and emotions have been through a lot. The world continued on so ease into it. As much as you hate to think so they got along without you for a few months....they can wait for you to catch up!

Am I different? I think so. I take more pleasure in the little things—the singing birds, playing cats, flowers growing in the yard, clouds floating by. I don't take for granted spending time with Tom. Those are precious times even if it's just sitting by each other silently.

I'm more conscientious about my health. I want to take better care of myself.

My thoughts and feelings:

Chapter 9

THE CO-SURVIVOR/CARETAKER'S PERSPECTIVE

The Susan B. Komen website, www.komen.org, describes a co-survivor as "…a treasured source of support and inspiration." Merriam-Webster Dictionary defines caretaker as "one that gives physical or emotional care and support".[4] On the cancer journey one needs a caretaker, someone who will provide physical and emotional support throughout. The following are thoughts from our co-survivors/caretakers.

Janice

Before I began this journey, "caretaker" was not a phrase in my vocabulary. I had only heard it in association with "cottage" as in 'he is the caretaker of our summer cottage.' It was an incredibly scary and honoring roller coaster ride to begin with my mom.

---

4   Merriam-Webster Dictionary

The night after the wedding in Iowa Mom came out of the motel bathroom and asked me to feel the lump. The first thought that popped into my head was, "My goodness, I haven't touched these since I was 6 months old and still nursing!" I remember the lump being large and hard. I tried to think of something encouraging and comforting to say, but for once in my life I could think of nothing to say. I think I knew, but I just couldn't or wouldn't say it out loud. I don't believe either of us slept much that night.

Sitting in the tiny cubicle waiting for the doctor to come and tell us the results of the biopsy seemed to take forever. I was torn, wanting to lighten the mood with witty repartee, yet knowing the gravity of the situation if the diagnosis was positive. I appreciated the doctors straightforwardness. He didn't beat around the bush when he said, "Mrs. Hulsey, you have cancer." I was anticipating it was indeed cancer and already had wet, but not drippy, eyes. When Mom said very calmly, serenely, "O.K., so what choices do I have?", the tears that were at the ready suddenly went in reverse. (By the way that kind of hurts.) Here I was sitting with the most incredibly strong woman I ever had the pleasure of knowing.

As I waited with Mom in the little pre-op room before her lumpectomy, she started to get sleepy. She said, "I don't know what is in that IV, but I'm getting sleepy." I had to be the one to break it to her that it was only a saline solution, they hadn't given her any drugs yet!

After the surgery it took her awhile to come out of the anesthesia. When we arrived home, my husband and brother decided it would be easier to get her in the house by using her office chair because it had wheels. As they wheeled her down the hallway, she insisted she could walk. They told her to lift her feet. With her feet in the air she kept saying, "no really, I can walk!"

As I put her in her pajamas and tucked her into bed to sleep off the rest of the anesthesia, my sisters went to the store to buy the extra support bras Mom would need during her recovery. What they had forgotten before they left was to get the size they needed to buy. As I looked through Mom's dresser drawer to find the correct size she roused enough to ask me what I was looking for, promptly told me and fell back asleep.

Later as I changed her dressing and very gently cleaned her drainage tubes, I was struck by how many times she had nursed <u>my</u> <u>wounds</u> and cared for <u>my</u> <u>needs</u>. I was finally able to do for her what she had done for me throughout the years.

A second time in the pre-op room, the doctor came in to talk with Mom. Again we had worn bandages over our breasts as we had the first time. As Dr. Roam was leaving, he poked his head back in to take another look at our bandages. He said, "oh yeah, you're the bandage family!"

This time the anesthesiologist eased up on the medication. Mom didn't take as long to recover. Once we were in the van, the first words out of her mouth were, "Let's go eat!"

Due to the frequency of our visits to the chemo treatment room you get to know the nurses quickly and pretty well. Somehow between Mom and I we managed to spill a soda or something at least once a visit. I would clean it up, so my backside was most recognizable. During one visit, one of the nurses was talking with me and said, "Oh, I almost didn't recognize you from this angle!"

As we left chemo treatments I half walked, half carried my normally very ladylike, sweet, modest mother to the vehicle. In a very loud, clear voice, she announced, "I've never been drunk before, but I think this must be what it feels like!"

The first time I saw Mom after her head was shaved, it struck me really hard. She has cancer. It's real. I was able to see what an incredibly perfect, round head she had! She was beautiful!

She usually only wore the turban around the house and as her hair started to slowly grow back, her head would sometimes itch under the turban. When she would scratch it through the turban, it inevitably would go askew. It was a sight, so without trying to laugh out loud, we would set it right.

Nancy, mom's neighbor, called me one night after she took mom to the emergency room thinking she had a heart attack. On the 30-minute trip to the hospital, I just kept saying to God, "No! You will not do this again! I cannot lose another parent so soon!" When I walked into the emergency room and saw her sitting up and smiling I thanked God for answering my prayers. This event happened to be on my birthday. Now while I liked to relive certain moments in my life, reliving the day of my birth in the hospital with Mom wasn't what I had in mind! We named her IV stand Fred. Of course he went with her everywhere. When she made a trip to the restroom, she would say, "come on, Fred." I spent two nights in the lounge chair in her hospital room. My husband finally came to pick me up at 11:00 PM so I could sleep in my own bed. I was back early the next morning.

I never thought I would see the day my God-fearing, Sunday School teaching, southern lady, modest Mother would get a tattoo! When it came time for radiation she had tattoos that served as guidelines for the radiation.

I went with Mom to have her port removed. The procedure was done in the doctor's office and I sat in the room as the surgeon removed it. Occasionally the surgeon would say "oops." After about the third "oops" I finally said, "no oops, no oops!" There wasn't a problem, Dr. Tabb just thought she was hurting Mom.

Tom

When one says the words of commitment in the wedding vows "...for better or for worse, for richer, for poorer, in sickness and in health, to love and to cherish; from this day forward until death do us part" they are merely words with meaning but devoid of definition. The defining begins as life happens. There is within a person an idea of how they think they should and will handle a crisis.

Until I heard the words from my wife's doctor "Mr. Carpenter, your wife has breast cancer," there was no way to be certain. Immediately the questions begin to swirl around in my head, 'Will she make it? Will she be disfigured? Will she be strong? Will I be strong? Will we have the faith and courage to get through? Will our relationship get stronger or will this drive us apart?'

I had no idea myself how to handle this crisis. My first notion was to discover all I could about breast cancer and its treatment. I wanted and needed to know what to expect. I am by nature a fixer. When I encounter a problem my first inclination is to assess the problem and then repair it. I needed information to plan out how we were going to handle the problem, how we would attack and defeat this enemy called cancer.

The information we received arrived sparingly. It trickled out slowly, little by little, day by day, appointment after appointment. It seemed weeks passed before we knew anything. When we finally learned all the information about the diagnosis and how treatment would proceed, I realized this was a situation I had no ability to fix and little or no experience to understand. I soon realized that my wife didn't need me to fix the problem. She had a team of doctors and professionals prepared and ready to take her through the entire treatment. What she needed from me was stability and support for a long journey; someone to walk close beside her when she was afraid, frustrated or weary. I needed to be the person she could come to for support and to feel secure and safe when the questions, the pain, and the fear overwhelmed her.

The experience was a physical, emotional and spiritual roller coaster ride. There was no need for extraordinary strength or wisdom. Just be available and willing to hold one another and to hold on together no matter what might come. There is truly strength in numbers, "...a cord of three strands is not easily broken," Ecclesiastes 4:12 (NIV) The strain can be intense but the power of two together is potent.

One task I learned quickly was to listen closely to doctors' and nurses' reports and explanations. I even began keeping notes during these sessions. Invariably we would find ourselves at home after an appointment trying to recall and sort out information. There is a vast amount of data to synthesize, future appointments and treatments to remember, diagnosis to pay attention to and medications with precise instructions, wound care and bandages that needed attention. The professionals do a tremendous job of explaining and instructing, but it is a huge amount of information hitting you all at once. This may be routine to medical personnel but it is all new to the patient.

Angelia was worried about my reaction to any possible breast removal or disfigurement, while I was concerned that I might forever lose my greatest treasure, my wife and best friend. I wasn't concerned with physical attributes; those things were trivial compared to losing her good health or her life! It wasn't trivial to her. She saw the removal of a breast as losing a precious part of her distinctiveness as a woman. After much discussion and assurance she finally was able to face any surgery and treatments without this fear. Fortunately losing her breast wasn't an issue she had to face.

The scope of her treatment was very personalized. We were assured many times by many people every treatment is geared to the individual. The warning was given to not be concerned if others told of different experiences. Each treatment is different and each person responds in various ways to their treatment.

Then came the trauma of hair loss. One thing that is almost universally experienced is hair loss during chemotherapy. Angelia was told that in the third week of chemo she would begin to lose her hair. She had an appointment with her oncologist about that time and she still wasn't losing her hair. The doctor commented perhaps she was one of the few who wouldn't lose her hair. This prospect pleased Angelia and gave her a bit of hope that she might avoid this drama.

The very next day I received a call and I knew something was wrong. As if on cue Angelia's hair had started coming out in clumps as she showered that morning. Previously we had ordered a wig and it was on standby. She had arranged with a hair stylist to simply cut her hair short rather than allow it to fall out. It was upsetting to both of us. She became emotional and cried, but then faced this new experience bravely.

It was at first unsettling to see her with no hair. As good as her wig matched in style and color, it just was not her real look to me. I never told her this (until this writing), but I could never really like the wig. As time passed, so did the shock of seeing her with no hair. I can't say I liked it but it never bothered me. I knew the hair did not change who she was, just how she looked. She was still the person I loved and hair can grow back.

One of the greatest benefits of facing this illness was all the great people and professionals who helped by expressing their sincere help. I could list numerous doctors, specialists, nurses, and social workers who at just the right time shared an encouraging word or made us laugh. These are precious memories of precious people from difficult days.

No one made more of an impression on me than the hair stylist who dealt with Angelia the day she began losing her hair. She was so sympathetic and accommodating that afternoon. She moved her chair to a private location in the shop. She first comforted Angelia and helped calm her down. Then she styled the wig and fixed it so it pleased Angelia and then very quietly and unceremoniously she removed the hair and helped her place the wig. It was her job and she had done it many times before, but she was so kind and gentle. She helped us get through a difficult day with dignity and grace. She was like so many others...a God-send!

Wearing the wig was very hot for Angelia in the Louisiana heat and humidity. She would often remove it while at home and place it near our front door in case we had visitors. On one such occasion she was at the door about to let our guests enter. I noticed she had forgotten to put on her wig. I pointed to her bald head and she laughed and rolled her eyes. Hurriedly, she scrambled to find it and put it on before shocking our unsuspecting guest. As traumatic as this experience was we found many occasions to laugh about it. Eventually it became just another accepted part of dealing with cancer.

There is an ongoing difficulty as a cancer survivor— it is a new normal of life. Once a person is diagnosed, goes successfully through treatment, and is finally declared cancer free, they face the constant fear that it will return. This isn't fair but it is back to the uncertainty of everyday life. A survivor doesn't receive a free pass, but an intensified sensitivity to unanswered questions and concerns. Aches, pains and other health issues are always suspect. A doctor visit, a check-up or a mammogram is never again normal because of the risk a test may come back positive for cancer or an X-ray may reveal a spot or blood work is suspicious. It is always unsettling until the all clear is verified by the results. These are always anxious times, but face these dilemmas as best you can without worry, discover all the information you can, and live everyday to its fullest extent.

I want to share a simple compilation of thoughts to assist a caregiver seeking beneficial ideas to provide effective care to those they love.

Be a researcher—Gather and share information with your patient about practical aspects of their treatment. You can help find answers to the questions they may not ask anyone else.

Be a coalition builder—Seek and encourage gathering a community of support for the patient and yourself. There are many organizations offering everything from practical to professional help for patients and their families.

Be a voice—Speak up when the patient can't or won't.

Be a listener—Accompany your patient to appointments

and consultations so you can be an additional set of ears. The information is often overwhelming and is given fast. Two sets of ears can hear and attain it better!

Be positive—Encourage the patient. There will be days you will have to be the influence to keep them hopeful and positive.

Be realistic—Take care not to expect more than is reasonable of yourself physically, emotionally, or mentally. Take care of yourself by eating right, resting and giving yourself a respite.

Be prepared to go the distance.

Jean

I've started a new journey. Not one I ever wanted to take. My oldest daughter, Angelia, has been diagnosed with breast cancer. The hard part is she's so far away—I live in Missouri, she lives in Louisiana.

Perhaps unconcsciously I prayed when I was diagnosed that none of my daughters or granddaughters would have to experience breast cancer. But this I know..... there is hope. Cancer is not a death sentence.

Now each day my mind tracks what she will be experiencing with knowledge of what she will live with for the next year. Through my prayers I can walk with her on her journey. Tears were always close to the surface even though I believed she had been trusted to the Lord. It's always harder when your child is the one hurting.

But I knew too Angelia had a good caretaker—her husband, Tom. He's my hero.

Because of the kindness of some of Angelia's friends I was able to spend three weeks, in the beginning (surgeries and treatments) to help with her care. I kept thinking, "how much do I help and yet allow Angelia her independence?" Walk with her but don't push. It was an untraveled way for us but one many others have traveled. It became a bonding experience for us.

Before going to be with Angelia, as I was reading my Bible one day, Psalm 91 spoke strongly to me. These verses became promises to me for Angelia.

Whoever dwells in the shelter of the Most High
　　will rest in the shadow of the Almighty.
I will say of the Lord, "He is my refuge and my fortress,
　　my God, in whom I trust."
Surely he will save you
　　from the fowler's snare
　　and from the deadly pestilence.
He will cover you with his feathers,
　　and under his wings you will find refuge;
　　his faithfulness will be your shield and rampart.
You will not fear the terror of night,

nor the arrow that flies by day,
nor the pestilence that stalks in the darkness,
    nor the plague that destroys at midday.
A thousand may fall at your side,
    ten thousand at your right hand,
    but it will not come near you.
You will only observe with your eyes
    and see the punishment of the wicked.
If you say, "The Lord is my refuge,"
    and you make the Most High your dwelling,
no harm will overtake you,
    no disaster will come near your tent.
For he will command his angels concerning you
    to guard you in all your ways;
they will lift you up in their hands,
    so that you will not strike your foot against a stone.
You will tread on the lion and the cobra;
    you will trample the great lion and the serpent.
"Because he loves me," says the Lord, "I will rescue him;
    I will protect him, for he acknowledges my name.
He will call on me, and I will answer him;
    I will be with him in trouble,
    I will deliver him and honor him.
With long life I will satisfy him
    and show him my salvation."

Psalm 91:1-16 (NIV)

My thoughts and feelings:

SCRIPTURES THAT ENCOURAGED US

Exodus 15:26

Numbers 6:24-28

Deuteronomy 31:8

Psalm 42:11

Psalm 55:22

Psalm 56:3

Psalm 61:2

Psalm 77:10-14

Psalm 91

Psalm 121:7

Psalm 139:17

Psalm 145:8-9

Psalm 147:3

Isaiah 26:3

Isaiah 55:8

Isaiah 61:3

Jeremiah 29:11-13

Jeremiah 31:25

Lamentations 3:22-24

Matthew 10:30-31

John 2:8-10

1 Corinthians 15:19

Philippians 2:13

Philippians 4:7

2 Timothy 4:7

1 Peter 3:15

EPILOGUE

When I (Angelia) was diagnosed with cancer I turned to my mom for answers, comfort and encouragement. I saw how she faced cancer and continued living life. It seemed to be an inconvenience more than anything. I thought that was how everyone dealt with cancer.

I was encouraged by friends, who received my prayer e-mails, to write a book. I remember sitting at a table with several women at my husband's workplace. Rhonda had just been diagnosed with breast cancer. Her friends grilled me about the whole process. They wanted to know what was going to happen to her and how they could help.

That's when I thought a book might be helpful to others. Who better to help write it but my mom! How I handled cancer I learned from her. Hopefully we can pass that on to others.

We continue to be cancer free! Routinely scheduled check-ups are a vital part of the survivor regiment. Though you go in with optimism you find yourself holding your breath mentally until you walk out of the cancer center with the words, 'everything is clear' ringing in your ears. Continue those check-ups and follow-up tests. Be diligent about mammograms and self-examinations. It's what saved our lives.

Jean no longer has to take "the little cancer pill" that she was told she'd be on the rest of her life. She continues her busy life—traveling, church, teaching, visiting family, reading. Her final word—"There is hope. Cancer is not an automatic death sentence. There can be victory."

Angelia will be finished taking Tamoxifen in 2015. She had double-knee replacement surgery six months after her final chemo treatment. Six weeks after that surgery (when the doctor released her to drive) she started a new job. Tom bought her a mandolin for her last birthday and she is learning to play it. They hope to soon take the cruise that was planned for her 50th birthday and 15th wedding anniversary but interrupted for a bout with cancer.

Cancer can become who you are because doctors' appointments and treatments are all consuming. That time will pass. Sometimes we forget we had breast cancer. We are reminded when we have to check the "yes" box under cancer on a medical form; we step out of the shower, look in the mirror and see the scars and radiation darkened skin; we have to look in the mirror to shave our armpit and put on deodorant because there is no feeling in our armpits. At that point it becomes one of the things we did, not who we are.

If you are reading this book as a survivor or co-survivor and have found it beneficial please pass it on. We are still amazed at the people we come across who declare "I'm a breast cancer survivor."

Repeat with us:

We are survivors!

Printed in Great Britain
by Amazon.co.uk, Ltd.,
Marston Gate.